W9-ARB-630

mornings with God:
daily Bible devotional for women

mornings with God: daily Bible devotional for women

365 Devotions to Inspire Your Day

Dr. INDIA LOGAN

ROCKRIDGE
PRESS

Unless otherwise indicated, all Scripture quotations are taken from the Holy Bible, New International Version®, NIV®. Copyright © 1973, 1978, 1984, 2011 by Biblica Inc.® Used by permission. All rights reserved worldwide. Scripture quotations marked (ESV) are taken from The Holy Bible, English Standard Version, copyright © 2001 by Crossway Bibles, a division of Good News Publishers. Used by permission. All rights reserved.

All other quoted material is in the public domain.

Copyright © 2022 by Rockridge Press

All rights reserved. No part of this publication may be reproduced, stored in a retrieval system, or transmitted in any form or by any means, electronic, mechanical, photocopying, recording, scanning, or otherwise without the prior written permission of the Publisher. Requests to the Publisher for permission should be addressed to the Permissions Department, Rockridge Press, 1955 Broadway, Suite 400, Oakland, CA 94612.

First Rockridge Press trade paperback edition 2022

Rockridge Press and the Rockridge Press logo are trademarks or registered trademarks of Callisto Media Inc. and/or its affiliates in the United States and other countries and may not be used without written permission.

For general information on our other products and services, please contact our Customer Care Department within the United States at (866) 744-2665, or outside the United States at (510) 253-0500.

Paperback ISBN: 978-1-63878-749-5 | eBook ISBN: 978-1-68539-341-0

Manufactured in the United States of America

Interior and Cover Designer: Lisa Forde
Art Producer: Maya Melenchuk
Editor: Brian Sweeting
Production Editor: Ellina Litmanovich
Production Manager: Jose Olivera

Author photo courtesy of Kenn Hobbes Photography

10 9 8 7 6 5 4 3 2 1 0

TO AUNT DEBBIE:
Thank you for teaching me to pray,
to read my Bible, and to
love God because He loves us.

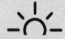

Introduction

Welcome to this yearlong devotional that I hope will inspire you to begin each day reflecting on God's word. This devotional requires only five minutes of your time a day and is perfect for the busy woman.

My name is India Logan. I am a doctor of education specializing in Christian ministries. I have devoted 10 years to ministering to women on social media, at events, and in church, but my story goes back further.

When I was six years old, I placed a tea set, a table, and one chair in the corner of my room and designated that area to God. During teatime with God, I would say that the chair was God's chair. No one was allowed to sit in the chair; in fact, I did not sit in the chair because, after all, it was God's chair.

The beautiful thing about this story is that no one was teaching me about God at that time in my life. How did I know that God needed a chair and that no one else sits on the throne but God? When people ask about my faith, I start with that story. I was not raised in a home that taught about Jesus or the Bible. I simply knew that He existed.

I experienced a lot of abuse growing up, so I grew to be angry and depressed. When I left home for undergrad in New York City, I was hot-tempered and unhealed from the childhood trauma. I could be found drinking at parties or in dance battles at clubs every weekend. During my junior year, I felt God calling me into a relationship with Him. I wanted to see change in my relationships and within myself. I was deep in the pit of shame, self-doubt, and depression. This tug at my heart felt like an invitation to live differently. I began taking 45-minute subway rides at 8:00 a.m. every Sunday to a small church in the Bronx. I began studying my Bible nonstop. I would go to sleep listening to sermons. I immersed myself in the text. The Bible changed my life. The promises living in the Bible, such as those found in 1 John 4:4, 2 Corinthians 5:17, and Matthew 6:14, pulled me out of the pit of shame and depression and into the light of forgiveness for myself and others.

I pray that my passion for the Bible inspires you. This devotional will teach you the Scripture and encourage you to apply it to your life. This devotional will encourage you. Each of the 365 entries includes Scripture and a devotional commentary to help you understand the Scripture. Full-page devotionals also include "Live Out the Word" prompts to help you reflect upon and apply the Scripture to your life. If you miss a day, simply pick up where you left off.

I pray you enjoy this devotional and that you have a fruitful experience.

1 | No More Shame in Christ

*Therefore, if anyone is in Christ, the new creation has
come: The old has gone, behold, the new is here!*

—2 CORINTHIANS 5:17

Do you ever find yourself carrying the weight of past mistakes and wearing the cloak of shame and guilt? This verse is your reminder that Jesus has redeemed you. Your mistakes do not inhibit you from having a relationship with God. Instead, your new identity in Christ connects you to righteousness rather than condemnation. God knows your past, present, and future mistakes and won't give up on you. God knows your beginning and your end and everything in between and loves you anyhow. Your shortcomings are no surprise to God. He calls you redeemed, renewed, and restored; you have been made new. You may not be able to alter your past, but you have the power to forgive yourself. Shame is the enemy's attempt to deceive you into believing that you are not deserving of love, grace, and forgiveness. But God deems you forgiven, worthy, and deserving of a good life.

You are free in Christ. Your mistakes do not separate you from the love of God, nor do they deem you unworthy. You are redeemed and loved.

Live Out the Word

What causes you to feel shame? Repeat 2 Corinthians 5:17 when you feel shame. Ask God for the grace to see yourself through His lens.

2 | Who You Are in Christ

I praise you because I am fearfully and wonderfully made; your works are wonderful; I know that full well.

—PSALM 139:14

God, Creator of the Universe, looked at the world and saw that the world needed you. A perfect God created you in His image. God is intentional and incapable of making mistakes. That means He intentionally created you, and you are not here by mistake. God deems you worthy, valuable, and loved. God calls you wonderful. In Hebrew, the word "fearfully" means "respectfully." Thus, you are a wonderful creation of God deserving of respect. Everything God does is for a divine purpose. You don't just have a purpose; you are purposed! Your identity is tied to a heavenly kingdom. You are coheirs with Jesus, meaning you are royalty. When your crown begins to tilt and feelings of being unworthy, undeserving, unloved, or unskilled surface, remember whose you are and where you come from. You are royalty. Fix your crown. You come from the very hands of the Creator of Heaven and Earth. No one on Earth is you, and that is a wonder to behold. You are unique, set apart, created divinely, and loved.

Live Out the Word

Journal about what being wonderful and deserving of respect means to you. Consider what God says about you. Review those truths frequently to increase personal confidence.

3 | Loving God Out Loud

If you love me, keep my commands.

—JOHN 14:15

Keeping God's commands reflects your love for God. Your actions may not always reflect obedience, but God knows your heart. Falling short does not mean that you do not love God, it means that you are human. The more time you spend with God, the more like Him you become. Time with God incites a natural desire to keep His commands. God will never command you to do something that you cannot. His orders are intended to bless and protect you while improving your life.

4 | Strengthen Your Relationship with God

We love because he first loved us.

—1 JOHN 4:19

God has always and will always love you. One of the highest expressions of love is sacrifice. God so desired a relationship with you that He sent His son to die on a cross for you so that your mistakes would not separate you from Him. To strengthen your relationship with God, seek to love Him the way He loved you, through sacrifice. Sacrifice personal time and read the Bible, because in many ways it is His love letter to you. Pray often and worship Him.

5 | Pray Boldly

> *Therefore I tell you, whatever you ask for in prayer,*
> *believe that you have received it, and it will be yours.*
>
> **—MARK 11:24**

Have you ever felt like God was not hearing your prayers?
God hears you, and He cares for you. Your prayers matter
to God. God wants you to make bold prayer requests. Bold
prayer requests let God know that you trust His capabilities.
When you pray, trust that God hears you, that He understands, and that He cares about your heart's desires. God
wants to deliver on His promises to you. Ask God for big
things; He is able. After all, we serve a big God.

6 | How to Keep the Momentum

> *I have fought the good fight, I have finished the race,*
> *I have kept the faith.*
>
> **—2 TIMOTHY 4:7**

Your efforts do not go unacknowledged. At God's appointed
time, you will walk into the abundance of God's blessings
for you. You are not invisible to God; you never will be. Keep
fighting the good fight. Understand that God bestows upon
you grace, power, and a willingness to succeed beyond
your wildest dreams. The seeds of greatness that live within
need your devotion and unwavering commitment. You can
and you will succeed. When you are teamed up with God,
you are destined to soar.

7 | Take That Leap of Faith

I can do all this through him who gives me strength.

—PHILIPPIANS 4:13

Paul learned to be content despite any circumstances. While we are often given this verse to encourage us to believe we can do anything, in context, Paul asserts that you can do all that God is calling you to do. Take that leap of faith to fulfill your calling. When natural circumstances do not appear favorable, trust that God will align the right people and opportunities, and He'll open doors. Do not allow unfavorable circumstances to dissuade you rather than challenge you. God is with you in everything.

8 | So Much Power in Forgiveness

Bear with each other and forgive one another if any of you has a grievance against someone. Forgive as the LORD forgave you.

—COLOSSIANS 3:13

God understands how hard it can be to forgive, but He also perceives that unforgiveness is disruptive. To deny forgiveness can trigger unhappiness, bitterness, and anger. God does not want us to live weighed down by other people's mistakes. God wants us to be free. Forgiveness offers freedom. Forgiveness is seldom deserved; it is something we must be gracious enough to offer. Avoid holding people hostage to a past they cannot change; instead, hold them accountable to better treatment. Move forward; you deserve to be free.

9 | You Were Created to Trust God

> *Trust in the LORD with all your heart and lean not on your own understanding; in all your ways submit to him, and he will make your paths straight.*

−PROVERBS 3:5−6

We often make plans and then include God rather than allowing God to be the decision maker over our lives. But trusting God means humbly accepting that He knows what is best for you and believing that His plan will come to fruition. Instead of planning for what you think your life should look like, submit your will to His. God wants His best for you. Trusting God empowers you to submit your plans to His. Trust God to be the executive decision maker over your life.

10 | Pray Confident Prayers

> *In him and through faith in him we may approach God with freedom and confidence.*

−EPHESIANS 3:12

Ephesians 3:12 is Paul's petition for confidence in His ministry. In the same way, you can confidently make your requests known unto God. Prayer is powerful; it is an outward declaration of your faith. Confident prayers reveal that you know who God is and what He has the power to do for you. You never have to be reluctant or timid in your prayers. Approach God confidently. God wants you to know that when you approach Him, He hearkens with His ears and heart unto your requests.

11 | Fearless 365

For I am the LORD *your God who takes hold of your right hand and says to you, Do not fear; I will help you.*

—ISAIAH 41:13

Fear is often rooted in our inability to control the outcome of past, present, or future events. God is with you, and He never wants you to fear. If you are afraid to do something that could be good, do it afraid. God never fears, so why should you? You are teamed up with Him; what better teammate could you have? Fear is a lie masquerading as truth. Fear attempts to deceive you into believing that you will fail, but let your faith outweigh fear.

12 | God Is a Promise Keeper

Being fully persuaded that God had power to do what he had promised.

—ROMANS 4:21

Abraham believed God for a long-awaited promise. In Abraham's waiting season, he continued to praise God. Abraham was persuaded that God had the power to do what He had promised. God's word is not void. He can and will fulfill His promises to you. Have you been waiting for God to fulfill a promise to you? Maybe you are praying for a successful pregnancy, a new job, or a healing miracle. God is an all-of-a-sudden God. He will show up for you.

13 | Hope in the Storm

But those who hope in the LORD will renew their strength. They will soar on wings like eagles; they will run and not grow weary, they will walk and not be faint.

—ISAIAH 40:31

While it can be difficult to remain hopeful in tough situations, Isaiah 40:31 is a reminder that when life feels unbearable, there is hope in the Lord. Isaiah gave this encouragement to the Israelites who were in distress from battling political oppression. In the same way, when you feel hopeless from the weight of uncontrollable circumstances, trust that God will scoop you up in His warm embrace and restore you. God will renew your faith, restore your hope, and replenish your strength. Eagles are powerful and protective. God provides you resilience and unwavering strength to withstand the storms of life. When a storm surfaces, eagles fly over the storm and soar above the chaos beneath them. Eagles are protective of their eaglets and strive to keep them safe. In the same way, God will cover you, protect you, and help you soar while the storm goes on beneath you. Storms can be turbulent, but there is stability, strength, and power in hoping in God. He is your safety net in the storm.

Live Out the Word

Write down how you can be more reliant upon God in your storms (for example: renewed faith, more trust). Ask Him to restore your hope.

14 | Waiting in Hopeful Expectation

> *Wait for the LORD; be strong and take heart*
> *and wait for the LORD.*
>
> **—PSALM 27:14**

While some of us are born with a high level of patience, the rest of us must train ourselves to be patient. Patience is the ability to wait with a positive outlook. Waiting can feel uncomfortable, but the beauty in waiting on God is that you are never waiting in vain. God's timing is different from yours, but it is perfect. Waiting on God builds character and strengthens our faith. Waiting on God means you want the best for your life. Rushing to make things happen rather than waiting can create problems. Psalm 27:14 twice reminds us to wait for the Lord. You are encouraged to be strong and to take heart. Waiting on God requires strength, the ability to trust God, and to be still. You have the power and the strength to wait in hopeful expectation for the promises of God. After all, He's never failed you before; why would He start now? When God delivers on His promises, He supersedes your expectations. Remember great things take time. God is never late.

Live Out the Word

What are you waiting for God to do in your life? Write a letter to God and ask Him for the grace to wait with a positive attitude.

15 | Never Alone

> *The LORD himself goes before you and will be*
> *with you; he will never leave you nor forsake you.*
> *Do not be afraid; do not be discouraged.*
>
> **—DEUTERONOMY 31:8**

God is with you in all things and in everything. He never leaves nor forsakes you. He loves you too much to allow you to go through life alone. He is devoted to you and committed to your life. God goes before you in the face of battle. He stands in front of you as your Protector, behind you as Defender and at your sides as Friend and Comforter. God is always with you. God has already won your life's battles.

16 | God's Ears Are Open

> *Then you will call on me and come and pray to me,*
> *and I will listen to you.*
>
> **—JEREMIAH 29:12**

When you call on God, He not only hears you; He listens to you. People may not always listen, understand, or care, but God does. When you call on the name of God, He hearkens His ears unto you, and He listens intently. God is eager to hear from you. God wants to know your heart's song and your spirit's cry; you are valuable. Always pray to God because He is listening.

17 | You Are Unconditionally Loved

> For God so loved the world that he gave his one
> and only Son, that whoever believes in him shall not
> perish but have eternal life.
>
> **—JOHN 3:16**

God sent His only son, Jesus, to die on a cross for you because He loves you. Before you were born, before you ever fell short, He covered you with His love. God loves you beyond your shortcomings and mistakes. He loves you unconditionally. You cannot work to earn God's love; He simply loves you. Nothing you do or have done will separate you from His love. People may leave you, hurt you, and stop loving you, but God will never stop loving you.

18 | Even Jesus Had Naysayers

> In your unfailing love, silence my enemies; destroy
> all my foes, for I am your servant.
>
> **—PSALM 143:12**

If Jesus had allowed the opinions, actions, and words of His enemies to distract Him, He would have delayed what God intended for His life. Although Jesus had naysayers and people who opposed Him, He was not moved by their disapproval of His life. Similarly, God wants you to focus on who He created you to be and your calling. Disregard those who oppose you and focus on those who celebrate you. God silences your enemies and dismantles their judgment of your good character.

19 | God Will Renew Your Strength

> *Come to me, all you who are weary and burdened,*
> *and I will give you rest.*
>
> **—MATTHEW 11:28**

When God created the universe and everything in it, He dedicated the seventh day to rest. In the same way, you not only have access to physical rest but spiritual rest. God desires for you to be fueled in mind, body, spirit, and soul. What a joy it is to know that we can seek God and find rest when we are burdened and weary. Rest is found in Jesus. Seek the Lord when you—your heart, spirit, and soul—feel heavy.

20 | The Battle Won't Last Always

> *God is our refuge and strength,*
> *an ever-present help in trouble.*
>
> **—PSALM 46:1**

God never promised a trouble-free life, but He promised that He would be present in your need. God loves you fiercely. He prepares a way for you when there seems to be no way. God covers you in love, grace, and mercy; He is your refuge, safety, and protection. God encamps Holy Angels around you. You are covered going in and coming out of battles. God protects you from dangers seen and unseen. He strengthens you in your battles and fights the battles you cannot.

21 | Faith, Hope, and Promises

> *Now faith is confidence in what we hope for and assurance about what we do not see.*
>
> **—HEBREWS 11:1**

Faith is not about what you can see in the natural; it is about what you can trust about the supernatural. Faith is trusting God to keep His promises. Consider all of the times that God has kept His promise to you. You can wait in confidence and hopeful expectation for God to keep His promises again. Faith is being assured that what God promises will manifest. Thank Him for what you do not see yet, and that will show Him your faith.

22 | Hearing God Speak

> *Call to me and I will answer you and tell you great and unsearchable things you do not know.*
>
> **—JEREMIAH 33:3**

God instructed Jeremiah to call on Him for answers during Jeremiah's hardship. In the same way, when you experience hardship in life, God desires to speak to you. God wants to speak life, hope, and wisdom over you. When you desire clarity, direction, or guidance from God, call on Him; He is willing and ready to offer you a word of encouragement. The Holy Spirit helps you to discern when God is speaking. You can be hopeful in knowing that God desires communication with you.

23 | Thank God

> *I will give thanks to you, LORD, with all my heart;*
> *I will tell of all your wonderful deeds.*
>
> **—PSALM 9:1**

David was a mighty warrior of battle who credited God for his victories. Consistently give God thanks, honor, glory, and praise. God keeps you safe, loves you unconditionally, provides a way out of no way, and deems you victorious through Him. Express thankfulness and gratitude for the gracious God who has kept you and loved you through everything. Testify to what God has done for you and through you. Speak boldly of His goodness and all that He does. Let others know Him through you.

24 | Reflect God's Love

> *And now these three remain: faith, hope and love.*
> *But the greatest of these is love.*
>
> **—1 CORINTHIANS 13:13**

The meaning behind Paul's instruction to the Corinthians was that spiritual gifts should not be void of love. Love should be the guiding force behind all that we do and perform. Faith in God and hope in His promises are valuable, but love is a manifestation of God. At His core, God is love. For God so loved us that He gave us love. In the same way, let all that you do be done in love. Let your existence be a reflection of God's love.

25 | God Is a Healer

*Heal me, LORD, and I will be healed; save me and
I will be saved, for you are the one I praise.*

—JEREMIAH 17:14

There is not a pain in this world that the Lord cannot heal.
Jeremiah was in distress and wanted to be healed and
saved from his sins and the sins of those around him. You
may battle with sin and temptation, but God can deliver
and redeem you. You *can* be healed from the pain *your* sin
caused *and* the pain from sin *others* caused. God can heal,
restore, and deliver you from *anything*. God can heal any
pain—physical, mental, spiritual, *and* emotional.

26 | You Can Overcome Anything

*You turned my wailing into dancing; you removed
my sackcloth and clothed me with joy.*

—PSALM 30:11

Sackcloth was worn in times of mourning and distress.
David relishes in the joy and gladness God provides in
exchange for mourning. Depression can feel like an end-
less cycle of sadness. Sadness is not foreign to God; He
sees you, He cares, and He understands. Elijah battled
depression, and God offered rest and food to comfort him.
Similarly, God will comfort you and provide for you in your
sadness. David sought refuge in the Lord and found himself
dancing. God turns your mourning to dancing.

27 | A Peace That Surpasses Worry

> *And the peace of God, which transcends all understanding, will guard your hearts and your minds in Christ Jesus.*
>
> **—PHILIPPIANS 4:7**

God provides supernatural peace that transcends all human understanding. While the world around you may tempt you to worry and encourage you to view things through a worrisome lens, God's accessible peace reigns supreme. Others will question your peace, and you can confidently say that God gave you peace in exchange for worry. Your life matters to God. He cares about what happens to you.

28 | You Are an Overcoming Survivor

> *No, in all these things we are more than conquerors through Him who loved us.*
>
> **—ROMANS 8:37**

Can tribulation separate us from the love of God? You may have been subjected to harm due to someone's sin and poor decisions, but you are not a victim; you are an overcoming survivor. Be mindful of the narrative you adopt about your life experiences. God does not call you a victim, He calls you a survivor. You are more than a conqueror. You have victory over your life's tribulations, pains, and offenses.

29 | Seeking God First

> *But seek first his kingdom and his righteousness,*
> *and all these things will be given to you as well.*
>
> **—MATTHEW 6:33**

God wants you to seek Him first because it shifts your focus to the provider rather than the provision. Whenever you have a need, seek to focus on God rather than the need. God wants you to be confident that He will supply all of your needs. Keeping your focus on God aligns your intentions with authenticity. Keeping your focus on God shows God that you trust Him to supply your needs. Focus on Him and everything else in your life will happen the way it should.

30 | Think on Things Above

> *Set your minds on things above, not on earthly things.*
>
> **—COLOSSIANS 3:2**

God perceives that the world is filled with things that could disrupt your peace, your heart, and your joy. The world is filled with influences that can stand in the way of your faith. God desires for you to lead a life that is pleasing to Him and fulfilling for you. Nothing in this world can fill you up like Jesus. Paul encouraged the Colossians to set their minds on things above because God provides peace, clarity, wisdom, and discernment. Keep your mind on God.

31 | The Beauty in Humility

For the LORD *takes delight in his people;*
he crowns the humble with victory.

—PSALM 149:4

God relishes those who reflect humility, particularly in a world where pride dominates many contexts. He crowns the humble with victory. It is delightful to know that you are crowned by the King in Heaven for your humility. Humility is a sign of security in who God made you without the need for external validation and approval. Humility is regard for others. Humility will open doors for you that no man can shut. God values and relishes the humble spirit of a believer.

32 | Be Thirsty for God

So, whether you eat or drink, or whatever you do,
do all to the glory of God.

—1 CORINTHIANS 10:31

Let all that you do glorify, honor, and praise God. When you make God first, He honors your efforts. Whatever you do, seek work as if working for God. God does not ask us for more than we have the capacity to commit to. He simply wants our firsts. First fruits are often applicable to tithes, though it can be applied to anything; your first thought, words, and time can be devoted to God. When you thirst for God, He replenishes, refuels, and restores you.

33 | Grace

*But to each one of us grace has been given
as Christ apportioned it.*

—EPHESIANS 4:7

Grace is a gift of kindness; it is free and unmerited. Grace is divine power working on your behalf to help you fulfill things you cannot fulfill on your own. What a joy it is to know that God distributes grace freely to you according to your needs. You are given a measure of grace to do all the things you have been called to do and to be who you were created to be. Grace is God's power working through you and for you.

34 | The Treasures of Your Heart

For where your treasure is, there your heart will be also.

—MATTHEW 6:21

Humans often fall in love with earthly possessions. Matthew instructs us to focus on God and the things of God. Your heart is important to God. Your heart reveals to God what is important to you. God examines our hearts. When your heart is pure and your intentions are genuine, your treasures in Heaven are great. When your heart is enveloped in God, it blesses the eternal you. While there is nothing wrong with enjoying Earth's treasures, remember that your treasures in Heaven are far greater.

35 | Abounding in Wisdom

*If any of you lacks wisdom, you should ask God,
who gives generously to all without
finding fault, and it will be given to you.*

—JAMES 1:5

Wisdom is using discernment to make informed decisions about your life. Wisdom protects you from making ill-informed decisions that can compromise your peace and joy. God cares for you; He wants you to make wise choices. God desires for you to have a life filled with love, peace, and joy. Since God's wisdom is far beyond our natural human rationalization, it is a blessing to have access to His divine wisdom. When you feel unsure, be confident in asking God for wisdom; He is generous.

36 | Be United in Christ

*How good and pleasant it is when God's people
live together in unity!*

—PSALM 133:1

God designed mankind for unity, connection, and relationship. In fact, God created Eve so that Adam would not be alone. God wanted His chosen people, the Jews, and the Gentiles to come together in their faith to worship Jesus. While unity can be hard, it is not without reason or reach. God perceives that a united body is stronger than a divided front. God relishes in unity because it promotes peace, joins common interests, and creates a stronger body of believers.

37 | You Are Just as Blessed

A heart at peace gives life to the body,
but envy rots the bones.

—PROVERBS 14:30

Envy is a result of comparing our realities to other people's highlight reels. It is commonplace to compare someone else's fruit to our own. It is vital to remember that we do not know what it cost to be that person. We do not perceive what it takes for people to be where they are. We do not know the private battles they fight and have fought. Their blessings are for them, and your blessings are for you. God has enough blessings to go around.

38 | Mindset in Relationships

In your relationships with one another,
have the same mindset as Christ Jesus.

—PHILIPPIANS 2:5

Paul encouraged the Philippians to adopt the humble mindset of Jesus in their relationships. The relationships that matter most to us require sacrifice, a little give-and-take, and unconditional love, all of which are rooted in humility. All relationships require intentional work and effort. Sometimes our relationships require that we humbly sacrifice our time, energy, and effort. In relationships, we must decide to agree to disagree, to pick and choose battles, and to think before we speak. Love commands humility.

39 | Singleness, Relationships, and Marriage

> *The LORD God said, "It is not good for the man to be alone. I will make a helper suitable for him."*
>
> **—GENESIS 2:18**

Whether you are single, in a relationship, or married, you are cherished. Singles, spend time with God and date yourself. The longest relationship you will ever have is the one you have with yourself. Mastering the ability to thrive alone assures you that connection is desirable, but it does not define you. Singleness is the time for unapologetic self-love. Singleness is not synonymous with aloneness. The same way Adam was with God in the garden prior to Eve's existence, God is with you, and desires one-on-one time with you. In His perfect time, He will provide a partner. If you are in a relationship, ask yourself if the relationship is a reflection of God's love for you. Does this person add to your relationship with God and fuel your Christian faith? If you are married, actively love on your partner the way they prefer to receive love. Seek to remember why you started. Keep God at the center of your marriage, allowing Him to be the source from which you pull strength, wisdom, and guidance.

Live Out the Word

Single: Practice self-care today. In a relationship: Jot down how your relationship fuels your faith walk. Partnered: Actively love on your partner with an unexpected gesture.

40 | Running to Jesus

You are my hiding place; you will protect me from
trouble and surround me with songs of deliverance.

—PSALM 32:7

You can seek refuge in God; He will protect you from things meant to harm you. He'll surround you with His grace and mercy. Your secrets, thoughts, and deepest sentiments are safe with God. To be hidden from the world is to be found with God. God desires alone time with you. The psalmist David wrote about the love, compassion, and safety found in being with God. God is not simply a hiding place; He is your hiding place.

41 | The Golden Rule

So in everything, do to others what you would have them
do to you, for this sums up the Law and the Prophets.

—MATTHEW 7:12

Kindness creates opportunities for valuable relationships and connections. Kindness can open doors and breed fruitful opportunities. You never know who you are sharing kindness with. The random person you complimented could be the CEO of the company you dream of working for. The woman you help at the grocery store could be struggling to feed her children. The beauty in kindness is that it is free. Being kind sets the tone for who you are and for what you want to be known for.

42 | Commitment and Trust for God

> *Commit your way to the LORD; trust in Him and He will do this.*
>
> **—PSALM 37:5**

Let God be God. Humans have the tendency to attempt to make things happen without God because waiting can feel unbearable. Other times we move before God because we do not trust that He hears us or cares about our desperation. Moving without God actually delays us. Attempting to do what only God can do can create a mess that we have to rely on God to fix. God cares for you; God hears you. God has plans for you, and His ways are good.

43 | There Is Room for Growth

> *Let the wise listen and add to their learning, and let the discerning get guidance.*
>
> **—PROVERBS 1:5**

Wisdom and guidance are powerful for those who are willing to grow and improve themselves. God offers you life experiences that contribute to your learning, growing, and discernment. Growth positively impacts our quality of life. Keep seeking knowledge, keep being willing to learn and listen to wise counsel. You never have to stop growing. The wise can add to their existing knowledge base. The highly skilled can advance in their skill sets. The knowledgeable can gain more insight. No one is without room for more growth.

44 | Power, Love, and Self-Discipline

> *For the Spirit God gave us does not make us timid,*
> *but gives us power, love and self-discipline.*
>
> **—2 TIMOTHY 1:7**

God gave us a spirit of power, love, and self-discipline. No matter what comes your way, you have the power to do hard things. You have the power to overcome obstacles, navigate life's complexities, and heal from past experiences. God gives you a spirit of love. You are brave enough to love yourself and to love others. You are powerful enough to love again after feeling unloved or mistreated. God gave us a spirit of self-discipline; you can overcome weaknesses and challenge yourself to greatness.

45 | Do It All Unto God

> *And whatever you do, in word or deed,*
> *do everything in the name of the LORD Jesus,*
> *giving thanks to God the Father through him.*
>
> **—COLOSSIANS 3:17**

Have you ever dreaded doing something? Maybe you struggle with a boss or regret a commitment you have made. Whatever it is, God wants you to work as if you are an ambassador for Christ and representative of Heaven. When you harbor an attitude of Christ that reflects a willingness to do your best, it reflects the heart of Jesus. Life is not always filled with moments we enjoy with the people we love, but we never have to allow our attitude to dictate our performance.

46 | You Are Salt and Light

> *You are the light of the world. A town built on a hill cannot be hidden.*
>
> **—MATTHEW 5:14**

Matthew describes the mission of Christians as being both salt and light. Salt adds substance to things. Salt is used for preserving food, and it is used for adding flavor. The metaphor of salt means when you share the love of Christ with those around you, you add substance. Your love for Christ can influence and impact the lives of others. Your Christian faith works to preserve your life and others'. Your faith adds flavor to the places you frequent. The world may not reflect God and His love, but you can. Light is used to illuminate darkness. Your faith lights up darkness and stands out in the midst of chaos. Light signifies deep insight and awareness. Thus, being the light means you teach others about the love of God and forgiveness through Jesus Christ. It is a privilege and an honor as a Christian to be the salt and the light of the world. Your faith is not something to be hidden but rather a belief to be shared and expressed with others.

Live Out the Word

Brainstorm ways you can actively model your faith and be the salt and the light at any upcoming events you plan to be present for.

47 | Help from the Holy Spirit

> *In the same way, the Spirit helps us in our weakness.*
> *We do not know what we ought to pray for, but the Spirit*
> *himself intercedes for us through wordless groans.*
>
> **—ROMANS 8:26**

Have you ever felt the kind of sadness that renders you speechless? Many of us lose words to describe our deepest feelings when our feelings are overwhelming. The Holy Spirit is your gift from Jesus. The Holy Spirit is a comforter. When you feel weak, sad, or unsure, you can rely on the Holy Spirit to comfort you and to speak to God for you. You may not have the right words, but the Holy Spirit understands. The Holy Spirit understands our pains and sentiments.

Live Out the Word

Sit with any heavy feelings and difficult emotions for a moment. Welcome the Holy Spirit into this space and ask God to fill you with comfort, love, and strength as you process these feelings.

48 | The Fruit of the Spirit

> *But the fruit of the Spirit is love, joy, peace, forbearance, kindness, goodness, faithfulness, gentleness and self-control. Against such things there is no law.*
>
> **—GALATIANS 5:22–23**

As a Christian, you have access to the precious gift of the Holy Spirit. In fact, the Holy Spirit lives within you and bears fruit! The fruit living within you is evidence of God's love for you, your relationship with Christ, and the gift of the Holy Spirit that was bestowed upon you. The fruit of the Spirit is love, joy, peace, patience, kindness, goodness, faithfulness, gentleness, and self-control. The fruits radiate outwardly when the Holy Spirit is alive and active within you. God wants you to experience authentic love. God wants you to embrace joy and radiate peace. God desires that you practice patience and kindness toward yourself and others. God believes that you can practice goodness and that you can be faithful to Him. You can be gentle with yourself and with others. You have the power to practice self-control and to do what is ultimately best for you, even when it is difficult. The fruit of the spirit is powerful because it contributes to your quality of life and impacts your life experiences.

Live Out the Word

What fruit are you readily able to see within yourself? Ask God to reveal to you how the Holy Spirit works within you.

49 | Test Them by Their Fruit

Thus, by their fruit you will recognize them.

—MATTHEW 7:20

Matthew warned against false prophets and inaccurate teaching. The encouragement Matthew gave was to test the fruit of people and things to protect yourself from ungodly experiences. You can discern what and who is deserving of your time, energy, and attention by examining their fruit. The fruit of wayward influences do not reflect the heart and mind of God. Test the fruit of people, things, and places. Examining the fruit of all things you spend time with can protect your heart, mind, and spirit from toxicity.

Live Out the Word

Take a moment to reflect and the people surrounding you in your daily life. How do they bear witness to the fruit of the Holy Spirit? Pray for guidance and discernment from the Lord in making decisions about how you commit time and energy to them.

50 | Motherhood

*Start children off on the way they should go, and even
when they are old they will not turn from it.*

—PROVERBS 22:6

If you are a mother or caretaker, God sees the hard effort
you apply while raising your children to be strong, indepen-
dent, and kind. Motherhood is an honor, but as with any
honorable role, it requires hard work, effort, and prayer. Ask
God for grace. God gives us His children to steward, teach,
love, and correct. Introduce your children to God, and He
will do the rest. What He starts in them, He will finish. He
gave you those specific kids because you are the best
person for the role. God is proud of how you lead them.
Single mothers: You are not alone. God is your helper. Married mothers: God sees your plate, and He offers you His
grace. Expectant mothers: You will be phenomenal. Future
mothers, mothers in waiting: God is a god of miracles. Stay
hopeful. Stepmothers: You are valuable. Empty nesters:
May your children always honor God and remember the love
you gave them. Mothers, be gentle with yourself. You are
doing your best. Forgive yourself and love as hard as you
know how.

Live Out the Word

Today I challenge you to pray over yourself and your children or the children in your life. Pray for the grace to parent
or care the way God would have you.

51 | God Is Merciful to You

*Let us then approach God's throne of grace with
confidence, so that we may receive mercy
and find grace to help us in our time of need.*

—HEBREWS 4:16

Mercy and grace are most meaningful when we hit rock
bottom. When you endure hardship, God desires that you
remember that you have access to Him. You may not feel
confident in approaching God, particularly when shame
creeps in, but God loves you too much to reject you. You
may not feel deserving of grace and mercy, but God looks
beyond your humanness.

52 | Modeling the Love of Jesus

*Finally, all of you, be like-minded, be sympathetic,
love one another, be compassionate and humble.*

—1 PETER 3:8

Share your faith, model sympathy, love others, exude
compassion, and remain humble. God cherishes the
moments you model His character. He calls Christians to
be like-minded in our faith because it breeds harmony and
unity. He asks for your sympathy and compassion toward
others because it is an extension of kindness. God calls you
to be compassionate and sympathetic because it exudes
love. When we work to radiate God's character, we bless
ourselves and others. It allows others to feel God's love
through us.

53 | Managing Your Emotions

> *Tremble and do not sin; when you are on your beds,*
> *search your hearts and be silent.*
>
> **—PSALM 4:4**

Have you ever gone to bed mad and awakened with clarity? Or maybe you have gone to bed mad and woke up angrier? Whatever the situation, anger does not have to rule you. Anger is often disappointment and devastation. Many people say " I am angry" rather than "I am hurt." People mask their pain with anger because anger feels like power and control while sadness feels like vulnerability. The reality is, being angry is not sinful; what you do with anger can be.

54 | God Is Working It Out

> *And we know that in all things God works for*
> *the good of those who love him, who*
> *have been called according to his purpose.*
>
> **—ROMANS 8:28**

Have you ever regretted a decision you made or the way things turned out in your life? God wants you to know that He works all things out for your good. You may view something you have done as the ultimate mistake, but God views mistakes as opportunities to learn, grow, and strengthen. God's power is not stunted by any decision you have made in this life. He can work anything out for your good. With God, you can still lead a beautiful life.

55 | Pray without Doubt

But when you ask, you must believe and not doubt,
because the one who doubts is like
a wave of the sea, blown and tossed by the wind.

—JAMES 1:6

Have you been praying for something that seems impossible? Doubt creeps in when things do not look favorable. Our thoughts can be as unpredictable as waves, tossed by winds and moving back and forth at varying speeds. Be still. Remain constant in faith and consistent in belief. Settle your spirit. God is working even when it does not feel like He is working. God aligns and orchestrates the right people and doors of opportunities for you.

56 | Have Courage

Be on your guard; stand firm in the faith;
be courageous; be strong.

—1 CORINTHIANS 16:13

This Scripture shows Paul instructing the Corinthians to be mindful of false teaching, to stand firm in faith, and to be courageous and strong. The Corinthians were struggling with worldly influences. In the same way, be mindful of anything attempting to attack your faith. Your faith empowers you. Your faith is the anchor you can pull strength from. Protect your faith. Things and people in the world may seek to tarnish the truth and promote lies, but keep your courage and remain strong.

57 | No Condemnation in Christ Jesus

> *For God did not send his Son into the world to condemn the world, but to save the world through him.*
>
> **—JOHN 3: 17**

Some people have been alienated and rejected because of their mistakes, but your Heavenly Father says you have purpose. No one on Earth can discredit what God creates. No one has the power to belittle your existence. Regardless of what society says about you, you are redeemed. God worked out your redemption through the blood of Jesus; never allow guilt to dismiss that truth. Guilt is an overwhelming feeling of remorse about a mistake you cannot fix. People may reject and condemn you, but God never will.

58 | Keep Up the Good Fight

> *Let us not become weary in doing good, for at the proper time we will reap a harvest if we do not give up.*
>
> **—GALATIANS 6:9**

Are you currently working toward a dream? Keep fighting the good fight. Your hard work and efforts are not in vain. What you have the capacity to envision, you have the capacity to experience. When the dream feels distant, remember that destinations symbolize the ability to arrive. Keep going. God does not give empty promises. You cannot fail at pursuing a God-given dream. You have the willpower, tenacity, and the ability to succeed. The world needs what God put in you. Keep up the good work.

59 | Thank God for Being God

The LORD has done great things for us; We are glad.

—PSALM 126:3

Pause and give thanks to God for all that He has done. Simply think back to all of the times God provided for you and was faithful to you. Remember when He healed and delivered you? Thank God for being God. He loves you more than anyone else on this Earth. He cares for you more than anyone else could. He has numbered your hairs and caught your tears. He is loyal to you. He keeps His promises to you.

60 | Embrace the Day

The LORD has done it this very day; let us rejoice today and be glad.

—PSALM 118:24

Rejoice in this new day gifted to you! Every day that God wakes you He is reminding you that He has renewed mercies for you and that there is still life left for you to live. Maybe this day is another chance to get something right, to work harder, to pursue a dream, or to adopt a new lifestyle. Whatever it is, today is a new opportunity. What will you make of it? Rejoice in gladness for the ability to do something that matters.

61 | Healthy Dynamics

If possible, so far as it depends on you,
live at peace with everyone.

—ROMANS 12:18

When we work to take the high road, agree to disagree, or pick and choose battles wisely, we cultivate peace in our lives. You have the ability to control your emotions, calculate wise responses, and practice listening. Relationships require our commitment to being our best self. Being our best self often requires deep reflection, time with God, and self-care. These golden tools will help to cultivate healthier relationship dynamics. When we work to be our best, we operate better in our relationships.

62 | Everlasting Word

Heaven and earth will pass away,
but my words will not pass away.

—MATTHEW 24:35

If you are waiting for a breakthrough, deliverance, healing, or a promise, know that God's Word is everlasting, unshakable, and unchangeable; His Word is an unbreakable pact between mankind and the Creator. God's Word is constant. His Word is consistent and unwavering. Always seek to study God's Word. The Word of God will encourage, bless, and inspire you. The Word is sure to remain the same. When life feels difficult and you feel unsettled within, rely on the unchangeable and always truthful Word of God.

63 | God's Gifts to You

For God's gifts and his call are irrevocable.

—ROMANS 11:29

God's promises to the forefathers withstood the unfaithfulness of the chosen people. The Israelites were disobedient, but God still graciously extended their gifts and callings. This is not an invitation to be unfaithful to God, it is a reminder that when you are unfaithful, God is unwavering. God gifts us with a calling that nothing can stand in the way of, not even ourselves. The call of God in your life is destined for you despite mistakes, shortcomings, and naysayers.

64 | Slow to Speak

My dear brothers and sisters, take note of this:
Everyone should be quick to listen,
slow to speak and slow to become angry.

—JAMES 1:19

Listening intently to God provides for discernment and direction. Listening in our relationships can lead to quality communication habits. Taking the time to listen can eliminate misunderstandings, diffuse dissension, and provide clarity. The ability to control our emotions takes time and comes with much patient practice. God desires that we control our emotions and work to be slower to anger. It is valuable to listen more, speak after much thought and consideration, and choose peace over anger. Similarly, our relationship with God can be strengthened with these practices.

65 | Rich in Spirit

Better the poor whose walk is blameless than the rich whose ways are perverse.

—PROVERBS 28:6

It is far better to be in good standing with God than to please society with inauthenticity. He examines our hearts. No earthly pleasure can fulfill the hearts, minds, and souls of mankind like God. When people are materially blessed but lack spiritual wealth, they can miss the joy of a relationship with God. Your genuine heart and pure intentions set you apart. It is far better to be spiritually aligned than it is to be spiritually bankrupt. The real blessings lie waiting in Heaven.

66 | Reject the Naysayers

But do this with gentleness and respect, keeping a clear conscience, so that those who speak maliciously against your good behavior in Christ may be ashamed of their slander.

—1 PETER 3:15–16

In life you will encounter people who view you inaccurately. Always remember that if you are doing your best to be a good person, those who speak maliciously against you will be put to shame. It is unfortunate when good people are under the discrediting rhetoric of others. You are more than their mean words and misconceptions. Keep your wits about you. Remember that God knows who you are. People may not understand you or perceive you correctly, but God sees and knows you intuitively.

67 | God Is Your Provider

*And God is able to bless you abundantly, so that in
all things at all times, having all that
you need, you will abound in every good work.*

—2 CORINTHIANS 9:8

We can be confident knowing that God is our provider. God provides for our needs, and He equips us to be givers. As Christians, we can be generous and cheerful givers. God blesses His children with what they need. God provides for His children so that they may abound in every good work. Paul encouraged the Philippians and reminded them that God desired for them to willingly help others. Christians serve a God who cares about their needs. God will always provide for you.

68 | Protect Your Heart

*Above all else, guard your heart, for everything
you do flows from it.*

—PROVERBS 4:23

Your heart plays a major role in how you live your life and is vital to your internal well-being. The decisions you make and the things you do often stem from what lives in your heart. What you expose your heart to, whether in relationships and interactions or in certain places, can either serve to fill or break your heart. To guard your heart simply means to protect it against negativity and toxicity. When you align your heart and its desires with God, it blesses you.

69 | God Can Restore Anything

> He asked me, "Son of man, can these bones live?"
> I said, "Sovereign LORD, you alone know."
>
> **—EZEKIEL 37:3**

Have you been asking God to restore, renew, or resurrect something? Maybe you are hoping for a relationship with a parent or child to be strengthened. Maybe you desire that your marriage be restored to peace and joy. Whatever it is, God can restore it. Despite the amount of time and the severity of the situation, God can restore it. God can make old things new. God cares about restoration because He desires unity among people. If it is God's will, your relationship can be restored.

70 | Even God Rested

> There remains, then, a Sabbath—rest for the people
> of God; for anyone who enters God's rest also
> rests from their works, just as God did from his.
>
> **—HEBREWS 4:9–10**

God created the universe and rested on the Sabbath day. If God rested, you, too, need rest. Whether you are working, schooling, homemaking, or an entrepreneur, rest is essential. Rest does not slow down productivity, rest increases productivity. Rest provides clarity of thought and replenished energy. Work will never be scarce, but your ability to perform at your best can be. Avoid working from an empty place. Resting is self-care. Taking care of yourself ensures that you are able to be your best self.

71 | Power in Prayer

> *Very early in the morning, while it was still dark,*
> *Jesus got up, left the house and went*
> *off to a solitary place, where he prayed.*
>
> **—MARK 1:35**

Even Jesus prayed. Jesus had a private prayer life with God. In the same way, carve out time to be intentional in your prayer time with God. Prayer is conversation with God. Maybe you will rise before the rest of the house or spend lunch at work with God, whatever you do, be sure to incorporate daily prayer into your life. The conversations you have with God are the most powerful forms of communication you will have. Prayer invites God into your life, heart, and mind.

72 | Cast Your Cares on God

> *Casting all your anxieties on him*
> *because he cares for you.*
>
> **—1 PETER 5:7**

Anxiety is worry about things out of one's control and fear of events with an unpredictable or unfavorable outcome. No matter the outcome, God is with you. He has not left you before, and He will not start now. Anxiety can surface from social interactions. God wants you to walk confidently in who you are in Him. Casting your cares on Him means giving Him your worries, fears, and concerns. God cares for you and wants His best for your life. He is with you.

73 | Who Can Stand Against You

> *What, then, shall we say in response to these things?*
> *If God is for us, who can be against us?*
>
> **—ROMANS 8:31**

Have you ever felt like people were against you? God wants you to know that no matter who stands against you, He will still stand up for you. If God is for you, no one can succeed at being against you. When people try to slander your name or speak ill of your character, trust God to defend you and fight on your behalf. No one can block what God has for you. In fact, God will bless you in the presence of your enemies.

74 | Honest Feedback Breeds Growth

> *Therefore each of you must put off falsehood*
> *and speak truthfully to your*
> *neighbor, for we are all members of one body.*
>
> **—EPHESIANS 4:25**

God designed the body of believers to be a family operating as one body. Unity among believers should offer a safe space for honest conversations. It is better to have a circle of accountability partners than it is to cultivate relationships with people who will appease you with lies rather than real truth. We should expect that our brothers and sisters will speak to us truthfully. The body of Christ should work together to edify one another, grow, and advance in our faith in Christ.

75 | You Are Free in Christ

Now the LORD is the Spirit, and where the Spirit of the LORD is, there is freedom.

—2 CORINTHIANS 3:17

Before you were walking with Christ, you may have been in the world operating as one lost and unaware of the depth of God's love. Maybe you battled addiction, lust, greed, or deceit. Whatever it is, the very blood of Jesus Christ sets you free. You are free in Christ. You are no longer bound by the weight of sin and shortcomings. You overpower and overcome your backslidings. You are not called by your sin; you are called a Child of God. You are free.

76 | God's Protection

I keep my eyes always on the LORD. With him at my right hand, I will not be shaken.

—PSALM 16:8

Having God as your right hand means you have an all-powerful force to be reckoned with on your team. David kept his eyes on the Lord, and God was at his right hand. When you focus your attention on God, everything that attempts to attack your peace and joy becomes less powerful in your mind. What you focus your attention on can either detract from your faith or build your faith. Be intentional and focus your eyes on God rather than the battles of your life.

77 | Keeping God Before Everything Else

He is before all things, and in him all things hold together.

—COLOSSIANS 1:17

Life can get hectic and feel overwhelming with goals, friendships, responsibilities, work assignments, business ventures, school, and trying to fit in rest and self-care. Keeping God first in all things creates balance, peace, and harmony in your life. Keeping God first means spending time with Him, praying, and reading the Bible and biblically backed devotionals. God can help you find ways to balance everything. God wants to lighten your workload. He will replenish your energy and refuel your strength. You are capable.

78 | God Is a Just God

"For this son of mine was dead and is alive again; he was lost and is found." So they began to celebrate.

—LUKE 15:24

If you are concerned about someone who is traveling down the wrong path, stay the course in prayer. They may not know God, but God knows them. God loves all of His children and cares for everyone's salvation. Keep the faith for that person alive. Either you will reach that person in due season or God will find another way to reach that person. You never know how close that person is to knowing God for themselves. Keep being the salt and light in their lives.

79 | God's Perfect Timing

> *There is a time for everything, and a season for every activity under the heavens.*
>
> **—ECCLESIASTES 3:1**

God designates things to manifest in your life at an appointed time. While waiting does not always feel good, you are never waiting in vain. God has big plans for you; His plans require time and divine orchestrating. God is not forgetting about you or His promises to you. In your waiting seasons, God is grooming, preparing, and readying you to receive the promises of your life. The most powerful moments of your life are not happenstance and serendipity but rather divine orchestration and manifestation.

80 | Solitude with Jesus

> *But Jesus often withdrew to lonely places and prayed.*
>
> **—LUKE 5:16**

Have you considered creating a private space for you and God? God desires time alone with you. Jesus withdrew to be alone with God. Imagine the busyness of Jesus. He still managed to break away from the crowds, the disciples, and those meaning Him harm to simply pray. Jesus set an example for every Christian that no matter how busy you are and how many people need you, time alone with God is vital. It is vital to your spiritual, physical, mental, and emotional well-being.

81 | Stay Easygoing

> *A gentle answer turns away wrath,*
> *but a harsh word stirs up anger.*
>
> **—PROVERBS 15:1**

Have you ever been tempted to respond hastily to a rude person? No shame here; we all have. Struggling to hold back a rude response is not a sin, but choosing to relinquish your power to them can be. You have the power to keep your peace. You may not always encounter the kindest people, but we can be the kind of people who provide insightful responses rather than abrasive reactions. A harsh word may further incite aggression, but a gentle answer diffuses hostile situations.

82 | Stay Diligent

> *I press on toward the goal to win the prize for which God*
> *has called me heavenward in Christ Jesus.*
>
> **—PHILIPPIANS 3:14**

Diligence is the consistent effort to work toward something valuable to you. Pressing on toward the goal means being persistent. If faced with setbacks, pick up where you left off, and push forward. Pressing on toward the goal to win the prize for which God has called you heavenward in Christ Jesus simply means doing the thing God has called you to do despite obstacles, disappointments, and moments of despair. God will never abandon you where He guided you to go. You can do this!

83 | Speak Life over Yourself

> *The tongue has the power of life and death,*
> *and those who love it will eat its fruit.*
>
> **—PROVERBS 18:21**

Thoughts are seeds. The thoughts you water with time and attention take root and grow, while inner rhetoric shapes external experiences and conversations. Your thoughts and words will either produce a harvest or grow weeds that destroy. Practice speaking hope, faith, and healing over yourself; positive self-talk fuels you. The words you speak can give life to your spirit or they can crush your spirit. If your inner rhetoric does not align with what God says about you, realign your words to match His.

84 | A Good Friend

> *Therefore encourage one another and build each other*
> *up, just as in fact you are doing.*
>
> **—1 THESSALONIANS 5:11**

Paul found that the Thessalonians were encouraging and edifying one another. In the same way, seek to harbor friendships that are encouraging and edifying. Having friendships that nourish your spirit through the Word of God is powerful. Biblical encouragement is conducive for faith building. Believers should remind each other of the goodness of God, particularly when tough seasons arise. God desires for us to have relationships and friendships with people who will remind us of how good God is and how faithful He is.

85 | Keep Calm; God's Got You

> *The LORD Himself will fight for you;*
> *you need only to be still.*
>
> **—EXODUS 14:14**

In the midst of the storms of life, you can find peace and calmness in God. Any storm going on around you never has to get to you. Remaining calm reflects your faith in God; faith in God moves Him to do the impossible. Stay calm while God fights for you. He has got your problems figured out. God is faithful. God wants you to trust Him in your toughest seasons because He has you covered, and He will never fail you. He never has.

86 | Thank God in Advance

> *Now faith is confidence in what we hope for and*
> *assurance about what we do not see.*
>
> **—HEBREWS 11:1**

No faith is required to believe in things we can see and physically touch. Faith is trusting God for what you do not see yet. Faith is believing God will provide for you when the cards are stacked against you. Faith is knowing that despite what the reality looks like, God is still able. Having confidence in what you hope for is relying on who God is and who He has been to you. Thank God for the things you do not see yet.

87 | What a Gracious God

> *For sin shall no longer be your master, because you are not under the law, but under grace.*
>
> **—ROMANS 6:14**

Any guilt, shame, and condemnation you feel is powerless. Those feelings lack the power to override what God says about you. God wants you to dominate these feelings and walk in the authority of freedom that comes from living in His grace. God extends freedom to the sinner and the saint. He wants you to know that there is not a single thing you have done that will eliminate the grace He has for you. Jesus has unmerited grace for you and your shortcomings.

88 | You Are Stronger than Temptation

> *Watch and pray so that you will not fall into temptation. The spirit is willing, but the flesh is weak.*
>
> **—MATTHEW 26:41**

Temptation is not a sin; succumbing to temptation is sin. You have the power to withstand temptation. You have the power to overcome wrongdoing. Sin corrupts good character and disrupts moral aptitude. God's grace is big enough to cover your sin. Thank God that He is more powerful than your sin. That same power lives within you. You can cast down sin by praying and reading the word. Sin can misalign your life from God's plan. Be mindful; interrupt any patterns of sin.

89 | Free from Sin

Then you will know the truth, and the
truth will set you free.

—JOHN 8:32

Jesus was speaking to those who were freely sinning and disregarding His truth. He wants you to know that the truth is where your freedom lies. You may stumble, you may fall, but you can be set free. The truth may be hard to accept or live by, but it liberates you from the weight of sin. God wants you to be free, so He gives you access to the truth. The freedom you have access to is unlike any other; it is freedom in Christ.

90 | A New Thing

See, I am doing a new thing! Now it springs up;
do you not perceive it? I am making a way in the
wilderness and streams in the wasteland.

—ISAIAH 43:19

God redeemed the Israelites and fulfilled promises to them despite their sin. Poor decisions and sins do not inhibit God from doing a new thing in your life. God is not debilitated by your life's happenings. God is still in control. When your life feels out of control, remember that God never loses control. We often grow weary in worry about the messes of our lives, but God is not incapable of giving you a fresh start. God's perfect plan can still manifest in your life.

91 | You Are God's Handiwork

For we are God's handiwork, created in
Christ Jesus to do good works, which God
prepared in advance for us to do.

—EPHESIANS 2:10

You were created by a perfect God. You were created from His hands. If you ever feel unsure, remember that God is not unsure about the greatness that is you. God is fully aware of your potential. Are you? Train yourself to view self-doubt as uncertainty about God's artwork. Do not doubt what God created. He believes in you. He is perfect, limitless, and intentional. This means you were created by a perfectly limitless God, who does everything with purpose. You are capable of good works.

92 | God Will Supply Your Needs

And my God will supply every need of yours according
to his riches in glory in Christ Jesus.

—PHILIPPIANS 4:19

Have you ever worried about how you would make ends meet, provide for your kids, or get provision? God wants you to know that He is a supplier and a multiplier. He will supply your needs. Though you may be tempted to worry, remember that God is a way maker, a promise keeper, a hope fulfiller, and a provider. God cares for you, and He cares about what you need in this lifetime. God provided in the past, and He will do it again.

93 | Giving God Praise

Worship the LORD with gladness; come before him with joyful songs.

—PSALM 100:2

Heaven will be an experience of continual praise to the Lord. It will be an experience far better than anything you have experienced on Earth. Every day is another chance to worship God with gladness. When life is great, praise God. When life feels tough, praise God anyways. God deserves praises in and out of good seasons. No matter what your life looks like, God is still good; He is still deserving of honor, glory, and praise. He desires to hear your voice from Heaven.

94 | Loving God Back

Love the LORD, all his faithful people!
The LORD preserves those who are true to him,
but the proud he pays back in full.

—PSALM 31:23

God thinks your voice is beautiful, and He loves praises from you. While giving God praise and worship, you exude your love for Him. It reminds Him of your love for Him and faith in Him. His love is unwavering and unchangeable, strive to give that back to Him. God does not forget to wake you up in the morning, and He never forgets to love you. Try diligently to love on God, to love Him out loud, and to be bold in your love for Him.

95 | Allowing God to Mold You

> *Show me your ways,* LORD, *teach me your paths.*
>
> **—PSALM 25:4**

Jesus's ways are perfect and Holy. We are not perfect, but we can ask Jesus to help us be more like Him. The more time we spend with God, the more our character becomes a reflection of Him. Praying, studying the Bible, and worshipping Him provide you with a deeper sense of God's character and awareness about what He says about you. Time with God helps us to adopt His ways and develop His heart's attitude. Reflecting Christlike characteristics can impact your quality of life.

96 | You Are a Capable Leader

> *After that, he poured water into a basin and began to wash his disciples' feet, drying them with the towel that was wrapped around him.*
>
> **—JOHN 13:5**

Jesus was a humble and loving servant leader. You can lead your children, your business, your clients, and the people you mentor lovingly and humbly. Leadership is about servitude. Jesus was the ultimate servant leader. Jesus humbly washed His disciples' feet before He was to die for mankind. He even served the disciple who would betray Him. Jesus desires for you to lead with love, serve people selflessly, and remain humble. The best leaders strive to meet their followers' needs with grace and humility.

97 | Serving without Complaints

> *Do everything without grumbling or arguing.*
>
> **—PHILIPPIANS 2:14**

Jesus never complained about the multitudes of people coming to Him for help. In the same way, whenever you are tempted to complain, sit back and imagine Jesus helping people. He was selfless and unrelenting. The people who you serve need you. Your unrelenting love and presence matter. The various hats we wear can require a lot from us. But God wants you to know that He has given you grace; you have the capacity to humbly and graciously help others. You can do this.

98 | Healthy Words, Thoughts, and Heart

> *May these words of my mouth and this meditation of my heart be pleasing in your sight, LORD, my Rock and my Redeemer.*
>
> **—PSALM 19:14**

Your words can be a reflection of what is on your mind and in your heart. You have the power to speak light, develop healthy thought patterns, and harbor positivity. God wants you to lead a healthy mental life. When you focus on positivity, you exude positivity. When we train our minds to redirect from negative thought patterns and think about the positives, we enhance our life experiences. Our words, thoughts, and heart posture matters. Choose them wisely.

99 | Focus and Trust for God

You will keep in perfect peace those whose minds are steadfast, because they trust in you.

—ISAIAH 26:3

Make the decision to focus on God more than anything else. Trust God more than you trust your finances. Trust God more than people. Focus on God more than you focus on self-doubt. God is faithful, loyal, and committed to you. He will always provide for you, be your true friend, and give you encouragement. He has never failed you, and He will not start now. When you keep your mind on God and trust Him relentlessly, He will keep you in perfect peace.

100 | You Are Set Apart

Every good and perfect gift is from above, coming down from the Father of the heavenly lights, who does not change like shifting shadows.

—JAMES 1:17

God intentionally set apart unique gifts and assigned them to you. There are wonderful gifts within you. In fact, you may not know what some of your gifts are yet. Every day that you are alive, you have a chance to explore the hidden gifts that God bestowed on you. The beauty in self-discovery is that you may find talents that impact the world. God foreknew you; He predestined you for greatness. He prepared you and your gifts in advance for you to fully enjoy.

101 | Redeemed, Restored, Starting Over

Brothers and sisters, I do not consider myself yet to have taken hold of it. But one thing I do: Forgetting what is behind and straining toward what is ahead.

—PHILIPPIANS 3:13

You can start a new career after a bad one, remarry after a divorce, meet the love of your life after being with the wrong person, and heal from it all. God can change your life for the better. God can lead you in a new direction to give you a fresh start. Whether it is a rough breakup, divorce, hardship, or consequences of sin, a fresh start is available to you. Your life is not over, and God is not done with you yet.

102 | Walking in Truth

It has given me great joy to find some of your children walking in the truth, just as the Father commanded us.

—2 JOHN 1:4

Jesus has called you to walk in truth. In order to be the light, you must be willing to walk in the truth of God's word, instruction, and direction. Walking in alignment with the truth is walking away from negativity. It requires sacrifice, commitment, and unwavering devotion. You are capable. You are powerful; you can do this. Being a Christian may not always be easy, but it is certainly worth the love, peace, joy, and freedom found in the lifestyle. You are God's light.

103 | Keep Your Eyes Focused

Let your eyes look straight ahead; fix your
gaze directly before you.

—PROVERBS 4:25

Pay attention to the things that distract you. Those things may be attacking your inner peace, joy, confidence, or destiny. God wants to protect your heart, mind, body, and soul. God cautions you so that you stay in alignment with His will for your life. God does not want you to be distracted or discouraged. Many things in the world can seek to interrupt what God wants for your life, but if you keep your eyes on Him, His plans will come to pass for you.

104 | God Stays the Same

Jesus Christ is the same yesterday and
today and forever.

—HEBREWS 13:8

God covers you in His love, wraps you in His mercy, and calls you redeemed and restored. Most important, God calls you His. His love does not falter in the face of your mistakes. His loyalty does not change even when yours has. His devotion and commitment to you does not waver. God is the same yesterday, today, and forevermore, and His grace is always available. His love never changes for you. God's grace and love are gifts to be cherished. Thank God for being Him.

105 | Pray and Believe Like Hannah

> *As she kept on praying to the LORD,*
> *Eli observed her mouth.*
>
> **—1 SAMUEL 1:12**

Actively trust God. When you show God that your faith is unwavering, it compels Him to move on your behalf. Consider the unwavering faith of Hannah, who waited years for a child. Hannah held on to her faith and prayed relentlessly for a child. In God's perfect time, she birthed Samuel and multiple children after him. Similarly, your faith moves God and releases your blessings.

106 | God's Already Won Your Battles

> *I have told you these things, so that in me you*
> *may have peace. In this world you will have trouble.*
> *But take heart! I have overcome the world.*
>
> **—JOHN 16:33**

God goes before you, fights your battles, sustains you through tough times and brings you through trials and tribulations. He delivers you. God is never too busy to be with you in the storms of life. The battles of your life are never more powerful than the God of your life. God is a problem solver. He knew which battles would come and how He'd see you through those battles. With God you are victorious in all things.

107 | Direction from God's Word

All Scripture is God-breathed and is useful for teaching, rebuking, correcting and training in righteousness.

—2 TIMOTHY 3:16

Receiving and giving Biblical insight is vital for believers. When the Bible is the source of wisdom, it sustains the soul and replenishes the spirit. You can find refuge in God's Word. You can find encouragement in the Bible. Keep learning and growing from the Bible. God's Word is a solid truth any believer can stand and rely on. In moments of confusion, despair, or need, the Bible provides direction, clarity, and insight. We can strengthen our discernment by relying on God's Word.

108 | God Wants You to Win

Jesus looked at them and said, "With man this is impossible, but with God all things are possible."

—MATTHEW 19:26

When moments of despair or feelings of hopelessness arise, remember why you started. Remember who you started for and who you started with. When you start with God, He prepares the way for you. When things feel out of reach, remember that with Him, all things are possible. Where God guides, He provides. God will never forget His promise to you. When you lose sight of the goal, remind yourself that you were created for greatness. You can accomplish anything with God. God wants to see you win!

109 | Responding Humbly to Conflict

But he gives us more grace. That is why Scripture says:
"God opposes the proud but shows favor to the humble."

—JAMES 4:6

We must remember that not everyone is doing inner work and trying to be their best selves. Let them see God in you. One way to ensure we harbor peaceful dynamics and healthy interactions is to master the art of keeping our peace and responding with humility. Remember, your peace is your power, so do not relinquish it to anyone. You are more powerful than negativity. Choose peace and remain kind.

110 | Rest from the Stress

After he had dismissed them, he went
up on a mountainside by himself to pray.
Later that night, he was there alone.

—MATTHEW 14:23

Even Jesus replenished with the Lord. Exhaustion can cause a depleted spirit. God wants you to know that time with Him can replenish your energy and provide you with peace. Despite how hectic life can get, one of the most powerful things you can do for yourself is create private time with God. After all, being able to manage being an employee, a mom, a sister, a friend, a wife, or a student is a reflection of God's grace and mercy. Spending time with Him can sharpen your perspective and calm your spirit.

111 | Lay Your Worries Down

> *Do not be anxious about anything, but in every situation, by prayer and petition, with thanksgiving, present your requests to God.*
>
> **—PHILIPPIANS 4:6**

Lay your worries at the foot of the cross and keep trusting. Do not lose hope; keep believing. God hears your prayers and cares as much as you do about what is occurring in your life. Keep fighting the good fight of faith, and pray diligently, without ceasing. Keep allowing God to love on you, mold you, direct you, and guide you. God has not forgotten about you, and He never will. Did you know that God does not have the capacity to stop loving you?

112 | Mind on God

> *He replied, "You of little faith, why are you so afraid?" Then he got up and rebuked the winds and the waves, and it was completely calm.*
>
> **—MATTHEW 8:26**

What you focus on will amplify. When you place too much attention on life's storms, they amplify in your mind and appear more dominant than they truly are. When you focus on God, He becomes bigger than your problems and your problems begin to feel smaller. Be mindful that God can and will deliver you, cover you, or carry you out of the storm. No problem that arises is meant to harm you, but it might test your faith in the Creator. Trust God.

113 | You Are Not Condemned

> *Therefore, there is now no condemnation for those who are in Christ Jesus.*
>
> **—ROMANS 8:1**

God calls you by name. He does not call you by your past; He does not view you through the lens of your sins and mistakes. God does not condemn you for your sin; He acquits you. In Christ, everything is made new, including you. Despite what you have been through, what you have seen, and all that you have done, you can live in true freedom. There is no sin that can bind you up and hold you captive. God's love freed you.

114 | Iron Sharpens Iron

> *As iron sharpens iron, so one person sharpens another.*
>
> **—PROVERBS 27:17**

One of the most effective ways to grow and advance is by cultivating healthy relationships. Harboring relationships with people who are willing to speak honestly to you is powerful. Friends who challenge you with the truth of God's word are necessary. Growth comes from frank feedback and honest conversations. The way to grow is to be open to learning, be willing to receive honest feedback, and apply solid feedback. Honest feedback breeds growth.

115 | Your Cup Will Overflow

You prepare a table before me in the presence of my enemies. You anoint my head with oil; my cup overflows.

—PSALM 23:5

God loves you so unconditionally that when people fail you, He still blesses you. God is not deterred by what others do or say against you. You may lose friends in the world, but you will always have a friend in God. What God wants to do in your life cannot be stopped by anyone or anything. God wants to fulfill His word and His promises to you. God will cause your cup to overflow in the presence of your enemies. God is for you.

116 | Be Courageous and Strong

Have I not commanded you? Be strong and courageous. Do not be afraid; do not be discouraged, for the LORD your God will be with you wherever you go.

—JOSHUA 1:9

God wants you to know that no matter what happens in your life, He is with you. He wants you to be bold, strong, and courageous in the face of your adversities. God will never leave you in anything alone. You do not serve a God who is unable to empathize, but rather one who is compassionate. God did not leave you nor forsake you before, and He will not start now. No matter the outcome, God loves you, you matter, and you are valuable.

117 | God Hears You

*This is the confidence we have in approaching God: that
if we ask anything according to his will, he hears us.*

—1 JOHN 5:14

There is power in keeping God first in your life. Giving God
your first words can impact the course and direction of your
day. Over time, keeping God first positively shapes your life.
God wants to hear from you. God desires to hear your voice.
Whatever you are hoping for in this season, pray about it.
Prayer is one-on-one time spent with God talking about the
things you are hoping for, afraid of, or concerned about.
When you pray, God listens and He cares.

118 | Another Day, Another Chance

*He who began a good work in you will carry it on to
completion until the day of Christ Jesus.*

—PHILIPPIANS 1:6

God is not confined by human realities. God can make
possible what appears to be impossible. God is not limited
or confined by natural reality. God is supernatural; He can
do all things. God can reawaken dreams within you. Do you
think your chance passed you by? So long as you are alive,
it is not too late to pursue the things you envision for yourself. You can still become what you imagined you would be.
Every day is another chance and a new opportunity.

119 | Never Lacking

And why do you worry about clothes? See how the flowers of the field grow. They do not labor or spin.

—MATTHEW 6:28

God is a provider and a supplier of our needs. God tends to the lilies of the field. How much more would He be willing to provide for your needs? God is mindful of you. God cares for your well-being. It pleases God to meet your needs. God did not create you to live a life in constant need. Think back to the times when God provided for you in your need. Whenever you are in need, remember those moments of faithfulness.

120 | Stand Strong Against Ridiculers

If the world hates you, keep in mind that it hated me first.

—JOHN 15:18

God sees and knows you intimately. You do not have to be understandable to everyone. You do not have to be accepted or appreciated by everyone. What you should always work to do is love yourself whether others do or not. Sometimes the greatest peace you can provide yourself is remaining unmoved by the thoughts, opinions, and words of others. Jesus was perfect and blameless, and yet mankind ridiculed Him. If they would do it to Him, who are we in comparison? Stay strong.

121 | God Sees Your Hard Work

> *Whatever you do, work at it with all your heart, as working for the LORD, not for human masters.*
>
> **—COLOSSIANS 3:23**

Are you working diligently but feel like you have not seen the fruit of your labor or have not received proper recognition? Work as if God is your boss. God sees you and perceives how hard you work to succeed. Too often we look for recognition or acknowledgment from people and struggle to feel valued, when God is who we should seek to impress. Celebrate your smallest strides. God is in Heaven rooting for you, cheering you on and celebrating your milestones.

122 | God Is Listening

> *God has surely listened and has heard my prayer.*
>
> **—PSALM 66:19**

Prayer is an outward declaration of your faith in God. Keeping your faith empowers you to believe in your hopes. When you waver in your faith, it can be difficult to see how God can turn things around for your good, but He certainly will. God works in His own way and on His own time. God's timing may not always make sense, but it is perfect. Whenever you feel your faith wavering, recount all the times God was faithful to you.

123 | Seeds of Greatness

I am the vine, you are the branches; he who abides in Me and I in him, he bears much fruit, for apart from Me you can do nothing.

—JOHN 15:5

With God, you can do anything. God gave you gifts that only you execute like you. When tempted to be discouraged by your abilities or a saturated field, trust that God makes room for you. God put seeds of greatness in you. Water your seeds with time, attention, and effort. Your gifts can bless others. Whether your gifts allow you to pursue a business venture, start a project, or assume a new role, you are qualified, approved, and equipped for greatness. You can do this.

124 | You Have the Capacity

Like newborn babies, crave pure spiritual milk, so that by it you may grow up in your salvation.

—1 PETER 2:2

God created you with the capacity to thrive. He created everyone with capacities to be their best selves. You have the capacity to grow, learn, and become wiser. You have the capacity to become all that God created you for. You have the capacity to see your life evolve and to watch God manifest beautiful blessings from your hard work. God enjoys when we seek to keep learning, growing, and expanding. Our humility in acknowledging we still have room to grow ultimately blesses us.

125 | God's Plans Are Good

> *"For I know the plans I have for you," declares the LORD, "plans to prosper you and not to harm you, plans to give you hope and a future."*
>
> **—JEREMIAH 29:11**

Even when you cannot understand His methods and ways, His plans ultimately work out for your good. You may not perceive what God is doing in your life, but you can always trust what He's doing. God never plans to harm you. His will is better than anything you can plan for yourself. God sees your heart's desires and seeks to fulfill the desires that align with His will for your life. God will never fail you or lead you astray because He never has.

126 | Relationships Matter: Keep the Peace

> *Be completely humble and gentle; be patient, bearing with one another in love.*
>
> **—EPHESIANS 4:2**

While none of us are perfect, God's unmerited grace and love has redeemed us and gives us a relationship with Him that cannot be eradicated. In the same way, God wants us to model love, patience, and forgiveness in our relationships. Relationships are valuable to God; that is why He desires for you to reconcile yours. While relationships may change after offenses, God desires that we practice humility and patience with one another, offer gentleness as a response to offense, and strive to maintain the peace.

127 | Every Promise Fulfilled

Not one of all the LORD's good promises to Israel failed;
every one was fulfilled.

—JOSHUA 21:45

God is not limited nor is He confined to human circumstances. You serve a supernatural God who can do the
unimaginable. God does not forget about you; God does
not forget His promises. Remind yourself of all the times
God has shown up and done something miraculous for you.
God is not done blessing you. Every day that there is breath
in your lungs, there is still time for God to bless you. Keep
believing, praising, and praying as you await the promises of God.

128 | You Matter Here on Earth

Even though I walk through the darkest valley,
I will fear no evil, for you are with me;
your rod and your staff, they comfort me.

—PSALM 23:4

When sadness surfaces, remember that there is still hope in
God. Your life is no mistake; you are no mistake. Everything
God created was intentional. He breathed life into your
nostrils and deemed you valuable. Greatness comes for
you. You are purposed and destined for a time such as this.
Your life is worthy of being cherished. When troubles arise,
remember that God is with you and there is not a battle
you can lose with God on your side. You are comforted
and loved.

129 | God Is Your Refuge

> *The* LORD *is good, a refuge in times of trouble.*
> *He cares for those who trust in him.*
>
> **—NAHUM 1:7**

What concerns you concerns God. What keeps you up at night matters to Him. What you think about is important to Him. God cares for you deeply. Your words, thoughts, and feelings matter to Him. God is an ever-present help in the time of your need. He desires communication and connection with you because He loves you. Seeking refuge in God serves to keep your faith and your relationship with Him strong. Rely on God; He is dependable and reliable. God is your lifelong teammate.

130 | God Protects and Defends You

> *Do not take revenge, my dear friends, but leave*
> *room for God's wrath, for it is written: "It is mine to*
> *avenge; I will repay," says the* LORD.
>
> **—ROMANS 12:19**

Being a servant of the Lord gives you freedom and confidence that God can and will fight your battles. God defends you against those who seek to harm you. He protects you from your enemies. It may feel like your enemies get away with doing harmful things, but God sees everything, and He is a just God. God is committed to protecting and defending His children. He will not allow you to be overcome with someone else's poor treatment. He will protect you.

131 | God Is Your Teammate

*He rescues me unharmed from the battle waged
against me, even though many oppose me.*

—PSALMS 55:18

Some battles are ours to fight with God, and others are
His to fight for us. When you have done all that you can
do, know that the battle is no longer yours; it is the Lord's.
God's hands are the best hands for your battles to be in;
God is on your side; He is your best teammate. Your battles
will not overpower you; you will prevail. You are protected,
covered, and loved by an omnipotent and omniscient God.
He will deliver you.

132 | Discerning the Voice of God

*My sheep listen to my voice; I know them,
and they follow me.*

—JOHN 10:27

It is commonplace to feel unsure about what God is saying to
you. To discern what God is saying to you, ask yourself if the
instruction brings overwhelming peace, if the word is biblically supported, and if it aligns with the character of God. It
is easier to discern and understand what God is saying to you
when you read the Bible consistently. The Bible is filled with
truths and promises God has made to you. The Bible also
reveals God's character and heart for you.

133 | Give God Your Burdens

For my yoke is easy and my burden is light.

—MATTHEW 11:30

God understands and acknowledges the various complexities that surface in life. Whether it be work, motherhood, marriage, or daily tasks, God understands, and He cares. Lay your burdens down at the foot of His cross, for His yoke is light and His burden is easy. You do not have to live life without rest from responsibilities and routines. You do not have to shoulder the weight alone. Calling out to God is the first step in relinquishing your burdens to Him and being replenished.

134 | God Is Not Confined

Great is our LORD and mighty in power;
his understanding has no limit.

—PSALM 147:5

We do not serve a God who is limited or confined to natural circumstances; we serve a supernatural God with unlimited capabilities. He is an all-of-a-sudden God with a good plan for your life. You serve a God that does not lie and whose word cannot come back void. God is mighty and powerful. God is a promise keeper, deliverer of His word, and a God of good intention. He has never failed you before, and He will not start now.

135 | Thankful for the Days

> *But I will sing of your strength, in the morning*
> *I will sing of your love; for you are*
> *my fortress, my refuge in times of trouble.*
>
> **—PSALM 59:16**

God created this day to be unique and set apart from the others. Find rest and reassurance today that God is your fortress and refuge. Every day that you are alive is God's divine way of saying that no matter what troubles come your way, your life is not over. There are blessings in the supernatural realm with your name attached to them that you have yet to see! Be thankful for the day. New days are gifts and reminders of God's loving mercy.

136 | A Faithful God

> *If we are faithless, he remains faithful,*
> *for he cannot disown himself.*
>
> **—2 TIMOTHY 2:13**

God is faithful to you in your valley lows and mountain highs. God has been faithful to you even when you have been unfaithful to Him. He loves you in your messiest seasons and your triumphant seasons. God has deemed you victorious in the face of your battles. God has restored your faith and delivered you from the pits of sadness, shame, and despair. In moments when you have felt defeated, you were still victorious in Christ. In every season, God delivers, redeems, and restores you.

137 | Lead with Love

> *Do everything in love.*
>
> **—1 CORINTHIANS 16:14**

Faith and hope are rooted in human beliefs about the Divine, while love is the Divine. Love is the basis and foundation for God's connection to us. He created us because He loved us, foreknew us, and desired to have a relationship with us. He so loved us that when man failed Him, He responded with the purest form of love. He so desired a relationship and connection with us that He sent His only Son to die. Lead your life the way God does, with love.

138 | God Will Replace Your Heart

> *I will give you a new heart and put a new spirit in you; I will remove from you your heart of stone and give you a heart of flesh.*
>
> **—EZEKIEL 36:26**

God can heal your broken heart and provide you internal peace. God can heal the one who harmed you and give them a change of heart. God can restore your love life. God can renew a right spirit within you and give you a new heart. He can replace a stony heart and make it flesh. This means He can take the hardness from hurt and pain out and soften your heart again to make it open and receptive to receiving love again.

139 | You Are Powerful and Capable

So we say with confidence, "The LORD is my helper; I will not be afraid. What can mere mortals do to me?"

—HEBREWS 13:6

You are more powerful and capable than you know. God perceives how powerful, resilient, and capable you are with Him. Walk in the authority of your identity in Christ. Believe boldly that you are more powerful than what has happened to you. Be bold in the awareness of what God says about you rather than what man says about you. You are not limited or confined to the world's perception of you. You are not limited to what you have experienced in this life.

140 | God Consoles You

When anxiety was great within me, your consolation brought me joy.

—PSALM 94:19

God wants you to give him your worries because He cares for you. The things that cause you anxiety are not more powerful than God. The things that keep you up at night are not more powerful than your faith. Faith offers consolation. God ensures that your life's problems do not overcome you. When life is tough and you are still smiling and leading with peace, people will question how, and you will confidently say, "My God consoles and comforts me while giving me peace."

141 | Eyes on God

For the LORD your God is a consuming fire, a jealous God.

—DEUTERONOMY 4:24

When humans lose sight of the blesser in pursuit of the blessing, they make the blessing more valuable than the blesser. We serve a jealous God who desires to be your only God and your main focus. God desires for your intentions to be genuine, your heart to be pure, and your motives to be aligned with His will. When you put God first and make Him your main focus, He perceives it as trust in who He is. Keep your eyes on the Blesser.

142 | Your Mind and Heart

Test me, LORD, and try me; examine my heart and my mind.

—PSALM 26:2

Your mind and heart are powerful. Your mind and heart affect your quality of life. Keeping your mind on God and having God in your heart can protect you from making the wrong decisions or dwelling on negativity. When you ask God to test your mind and your heart, be prepared to see positive shifts and changes that evoke peace. The world may contribute to thoughts of doubt, shame, lust, and negativity, but God can shift your heart and mind to things that offer peace.

143 | Committing Your Life to God

> *Love the* LORD *your God with all your heart and with all your soul and with all your mind.*
>
> **—MATTHEW 22:37**

God does not ask for anything but love: love for Him, yourself, and others. Your love and commitment is a beautiful way to express gratitude for God. God simply wants you to devote your life to Him because it ultimately improves and enhances your life. God does not waver in His love and commitment to you. Committing yourself to God works for your good. Your life will not be void of trial, but it will be overflowing with love, peace, joy, and harmony.

144 | God Gives You Peace

> *Now may the* LORD *of peace himself give you peace at all times in every way. The* LORD *be with you all.*
>
> **—2 THESSALONIANS 3:16**

Living a balanced life provides peace. Often, accessing peace means eliminating distractions and spending quiet time with God. God desires time with you because He is the source of your strength. Make time for God. He woke you up and provided for you as He always does. Even in tough seasons, God is faithful. God provides divine peace. His peace is sustenance for the soul; His peace offers balance in the midst of chaos. God wants you to access peace, clarity, and wisdom.

145 | Citizenship from Heaven

For our citizenship is in heaven, from which also we
eagerly wait for a Savior, the LORD Jesus Christ.

—PHILIPPIANS 3:20

Your identity is in Christ, and your citizenship is in Heaven. Earth is not our permanent home. What Earth offers cannot compare to the beauty that awaits you in Heaven. Earth and everything in it will pass away, but God is eternal. What God has for you in Heaven is unable to be corrupted or destroyed. Focus your heart on the matters above rather than the temporal luxuries of Earth. Earthly treasures are fleeting, but Heaven's treasures are everlasting. Align your heart with heavenly desires.

146 | At God's Appointed Time

Humble yourselves, therefore, under God's mighty hand,
that he may lift you up in due time.

—1 PETER 5:6

You serve an intentional God who is precise and meticulous. When things manifest in your life in perfect timing and peacefully, it is God. God knows how and when things need to occur in your life. God desires to bless you in a manner that declares His goodness over your life. God wants to bless you in a way that makes others say, "You know that was God." The timing of your life is not accidental; it is intentional. Keep trusting while you wait.

147 | Harboring Peaceful and Positive Relationships

Blessed are the peacemakers, for they will be called children of God.

—MATTHEW 5:9

Peace, love, and joy are what your heart deserves. While tough situations can infuse bitterness, dissension, and disruption in your life, God does not want you to lead a life filled with chaos and toxicity. Protect your heart from relationship dynamics, friendships, and connections that reflect negativity, chaos, and dissension. Seek to harbor positive connections and cultivate peaceful relationships. Peaceful connections encourage a healthy lifestyle. Cultivate healthy relationships by harboring inner peace through self-care, asking God's discernment, and placing Him first.

148 | God Will Bless You

The LORD bless you and keep you.

—NUMBERS 6:24

God does not run out of blessings. Maybe you are awaiting a blessing that someone else has already received. Your timetable will not look like their timetable. At God's appointed time, you will reap your blessings. Do not lose hope. God has handpicked blessings for you. God wants you to keep a peaceful heart. Your heart at peace looks like contentment with the timing of your life, appreciation for your life's journey, and gratitude for your present and future blessings. God plans to bless you.

149 | Your Debt Is Paid

> *I, even I, am he who blots out your transgressions,*
> *for my own sake, and remembers your sins no more.*
>
> **—ISAIAH 43:25**

God did not send Jesus to die on a cross to condemn you, but to save you. There is no mistake that God does not cover with His love. You are human, you are imperfect, and you are loved. You may not be able to change your mistakes, but you can accept that God wipes your slate clean, renews your spirit, restores your faith, and redeems you. The blood of Jesus Christ covers you, and God loves you unconditionally.

150 | Peaceful Connections with Others

> *When pride comes, then comes disgrace,*
> *but with humility comes wisdom.*
>
> **—PROVERBS 11:2**

Our greatest duty to God and to others is to love. Jesus commanded us to love God, ourselves, and others. Valuable relationships require a willingness to humbly love with words and actions. Loving like Jesus requires us to adopt humility as our default behavior and as a first response in our relationships. Humility is casting down abrasive thoughts and behaviors as an attempt to maintain peace and love more intentionally. Humility is accepting your loved ones for who they are, while valuing your differences.

151 | God's Powerful Love for You

> *There is no fear in love. But perfect love drives out fear, because fear has to do with punishment. The one who fears is not made perfect in love.*
>
> **—1 JOHN 4:18**

Fear has no home in you. Let the love that God offers flow through you, fill you, and cover you. Let the love that God offers heal you. You have the power to eliminate poor habits or disruptive tendencies that compromise peace and joy from freely flowing to you. God wants you to live a life that radiates power, love, and a sound mind. When you fall short or experience tough seasons, God's love will cover you, protect you, and redeem you.

152 | Never Too Messy for God

> *Then I said, "Here I am, I have come—it is written about me in the scroll. I desire to do your will, my God; your law is within my heart."*
>
> **—PSALM 40:7**

Have you ever felt like you and your life were messy beyond repair? God will turn your messes into a powerful message. God is not confined by any poor decision; He still calls you His child. God will take your mistakes and use them to manifest positivity in your life. No matter the circumstances, God is still God, and you are still His. God can and will deliver you from the trenches of sin and shame. God can and will cover your wrongdoings with His love.

153 | Holy Spirit Guidance

> *And I will put my Spirit in you and move you to follow my decrees and be careful to keep my laws.*
>
> **—EZEKIEL 36:27**

The Holy Spirit provides grace and encouragement to help you keep God's commands. The commands for obedience, patience, peace, unity, humility, and love benefit you. The benefit of obedience is blessing, the benefit of patience is perseverance, the benefit of peace is harmony, the benefit of unity is connection, the benefit of humility is divine elevation, and the benefit of love is relationships. God wants His very best for you, so He requires your best efforts.

154 | Enough Kindness to Go Around

> *Those who are kind benefit themselves, but the cruel bring ruin on themselves.*
>
> **—PROVERBS 11:17**

Kindness reflects God's character. Choosing kindness allows God to love people through you. You never know why God aligns your path with certain people. Choose kindness because you may not perceive what someone is fighting through. God will put people in your path because He trusts that you will give them the kindness they need in their lives. In the same way, there may be moments in time where God purposely orchestrates for you to meet a kind person when you need it most.

155 | The Power of Your Faith

> *Because you know that the testing of your faith produces perseverance.*
>
> **—JAMES 1:3**

Continue to be the light of this world and exude strength. Be courageous and stand for what you believe in. Be strong against anything that seeks to compromise your identity in Christ. Your faith illuminates darkness. Your faith contributes to your internal growth. The impacts and influences of nonsupportive environments may attempt to muddy your faith, but stand firm. Keep your faith as a solid foundation and a pillar of strength in these moments. Be courageous in moments when your faith is challenged.

156 | God Will Give You Wisdom

> *For the LORD gives wisdom; from his mouth come knowledge and understanding.*
>
> **—PROVERBS 2:6**

God gives wisdom generously without faulting us for the things we did not know. Have you ever questioned what job to take, what program to study in school, or what parental advice to offer your kids? If you ever feel lost or uncertain about the matters of your life, God desires that you go to Him. He provides discernment, direction, and clarity. You can ask God, who freely and generously offers you His wisdom. The wisest decisions are made with God.

157 | God Is Your Shield

The LORD is my rock and my fortress and my deliverer,
My God, my rock, in whom I take refuge; My shield and
the horn of my salvation, my stronghold.

—PSALM 18:2

It is powerful to know that you can go to God, and He will shield you from the world. God is the one you go to to protect yourself from negative impacts. There are moments in our lives when we seek to be alone with God and away from the noise and chaos. There is peace, quietness, and stillness found in being with God. In these still, quiet moments, we can speak to God freely and hear Him clearly. He is the One with whom you can seek refuge, safety, and peace.

158 | God Is Gracious, Merciful, and Loving

You, LORD, are forgiving and good, abounding
in love to all who call to you.

—PSALM 86:5

God is devoted to you. God is kind, gentle, and loving toward you. God does not hold you hostage to your mistakes. He extends grace and mercy to you. He looks at you in awe. God wants His best for you. God studies your heart. When people leave, God stays. He loves you no matter what. When people harm and mistreat you, God comforts you, celebrates your wins, and looks for ways to bless you. Thank God; He has been good to you.

159 | Trusting God Through Everything

> *They will have no fear of bad news; their hearts are steadfast, trusting in the LORD.*
>
> **—PSALM 112:7**

Trust God through every trial, tribulation, waiting season, and uncertainty. When God closes a door, He's protecting you. When God does not open a door, He has something better in mind for you. Everything God does for you revolves around His superior will and His divine protection. You may not immediately perceive why God allows certain hardships, but with time comes appreciation for His omniscience. Thank God for building resilience in you and for protecting you. God is faithful, loyal, and committed to you. Trust Him, always.

160 | Gentle Words

> *The soothing tongue is a tree of life, but a perverse tongue crushes the spirit.*
>
> **—PROVERBS 15:4**

Your words can encourage you or discourage you. Be mindful of how you speak to yourself and how you speak about yourself. Your words can either produce confidence or dismantle your confidence. The words you speak can motivate you to pursue dreams and to believe in yourself or they can dissuade you from pursuing your calling. Your words affect your life. Seek to align your words with what God says about you. You are chosen, you are gifted, you are valuable, and you are loved.

161 | The Power of God's Word

The grass withers and the flowers fall, but the word of our God endures forever.

—ISAIAH 40:8

God does not authorize empty promises and baseless words of encouragement. You can rely on the truths, wisdom, and direction garnered from God's Word. The Word of God is uncorruptible; the Word is powerful. You can trust God's Word. His Word will never come back void. God is supernatural and unlike people, He does not go back on His Word or waver in thought. God is consistent in His character and in His Word. God is reliable. You can trust Him to be faithful.

162 | Keep Being the Light

In the same way, let your light shine before others, so that they may see your good works and give glory to your Father who is in heaven.

—MATTHEW 5:16

God entrusts you with being the salt and light in dark places. Honoring God with your work ethic is an outward declaration of gratitude for the opportunity to do something impactful. Maybe your work is important but the people you work with are difficult. Remember that if you shift your attitude to working as if you are working as an ambassador of Heaven under the direction of God, it can reframe your approach and in turn yield some strong responses. Continue to be the light.

163 | Harmony in the Body of Christ

Let us therefore make every effort to do what leads to peace and to mutual edification.

—ROMANS 14:19

He desires for His children to encourage one another and to help each other. When fellow brothers and sisters unite, it creates for a harmonious experience. Unity creates an unshakeable bond that radiates peace, love, and growth in Christ. Being united strengthens a body of believers in their faith. Strong faith provides a solid foundation to stand and rely on. When life gets tough, having a body of believers to pray for you and encourage you is invaluable. Unity is a valuable bond that can provide growth in faith.

164 | Rest Is Vital

In vain you rise early and stay up late, toiling for food to eat—for he grants sleep to those he loves.

—PSALM 127:2

Do you ever feel guilty for needing rest and when you try to rest you simply cannot? When we neglect our need for rest, we experience burnout from the things we love. We can begin to resent what we love because of burnout. God provides rest for those who are willing to enter into rest. What a joy it is to know that we can enter into His rest. In God, we have access to a renewed mind and spirit with replenished energy.

165 | God Is Compassionate

> *Then the* LORD *your God will restore your fortunes
> and have compassion on you and gather you again
> from all the nations where he scattered you.*

—DEUTERONOMY 30:3

No one and nothing can stand in the way of what God wants to do in your life. God has compassion for you. Poor decisions can delay when you access blessings, hence the Israelites and their struggle with obedience to God, but what God promises can still come to fruition. The Israelites were restored after being exiled, and God still blessed them. Your mistakes cannot overpower God. It is a blessing to know that we cannot stand in the way of a supernatural God's plans.

166 | God Is Mindful of You

> *What is mankind that you are mindful of them,
> human beings that you care for them?*

—PSALM 8:4

You are never forgotten. God cares for you; He knows your heart's desires. God hears your prayers. He knows your concerns, worries, doubts, and frustrations. Trust God to be present for you. He is mindful of you. God looks for ways to bless you. He moves mountains for you. Trusting God activates your faith and changes things. God can flip the script of your life. Pray and believe. Trust that He has heard you; He is working on your behalf; and He cares for you.

167 | God Is Working Through You

> *Now then go, and I, even I, will be with your mouth,*
> *and teach you what you are to say.*
>
> **—EXODUS 4:12**

Moses was fearful because of the calling on his life, but God reassured Moses that He would be with him. When God gives us visions that are bigger than ourselves, we often fear the journey. It's important to remember that we serve a fearless God that never fails. We never have to rely on our own capacity to do great because we have God. God teams up with us and ensures our success and victory. Let your work reflect the power of God in your life.

168 | Unconditional Mercy

> *When he saw the crowds, he had compassion*
> *on them, because they were harassed and helpless,*
> *like sheep without a shepherd.*
>
> **—MATTHEW 9:36**

Forgiveness and compassion are facets of God's mercy, unconditional love, and unmerited favor. You may not feel deserving of second chances, mercy, or grace, but your feelings do not dictate what God sees in you. God does not consider all is lost when you fall short or struggle. God has compassion, and He sees the best in you. God wants you to approach His throne of grace confidently, without fear of how He perceives you. God provides mercy and grace in your time of need.

169 | Being a Jesus Follower

> *By this everyone will know that you are my disciples,*
> *if you love one another.*
>
> **—JOHN 13:35**

Your commitment to being a follower of Christ is the most powerful commitment you will ever make. Your Christian identity sets you apart from the world. Committing to Jesus and identifying as His follower means you vow to humbly love others, view them through an empathetic lens, and offer compassion. The most powerful thing you can do for people is model the love of Christ. When you are a reflection of Him, it enhances the atmosphere you dwell in. Your presence shifts the room.

170 | The Power to Control Emotions

> *"In your anger do not sin": Do not let the sun*
> *go down while you are still angry.*
>
> **—EPHESIANS 4:26**

Sinning in our anger authorizes anger to control us. You have the power to control your responses. God does not require perfection from you, He simply knows what you have the power to handle. You are strong enough to be angry and remain sinless. There is power in taking time to think and process a situation. Thinking before responding gives our minds and bodies the chance to calm down, assess the situation, and respond maturely rather than reacting in sin. When we are quiet, God speaks.

171 | God Sees Your Heart

*Be still before the LORD and wait patiently for him;
do not fret when people succeed in their
ways, when they carry out their wicked schemes.*

—PSALM 37:7

It can be difficult to feel like you are working hard to be a good person when there are people around you who are not well-intentioned but appear to be blessed. Be mindful that God sees everything, and He is omniscient. He sees your heart and knows your intentions. Stay committed. God sees that you are authentic. Living in alignment with God is a far more blessed experience. Having a genuine heart with pure intentions is what sets you apart from poor life experiences.

172 | Believe in Your Prayers

*If you believe, you will receive whatever
you ask for in prayer.*

—MATTHEW 21:22

Prayer is an open line of communication with God. Be confident in your prayers. Confident prayers show God that you believe that He is listening and that He cares. God can and will do big things for you. God is a good father who has always been there, wants His best for you, and loves you unconditionally. You are His child, and in this you can be confident. You never have to fear that God will push you away or disregard your heart's message.

173 | Seeking God Daily Is Love

> *You will seek me and find me when you seek*
> *me with all your heart.*
>
> **—JEREMIAH 29:13**

Time is a powerful expression of love. God simply desires time with you. A relationship with God is not like any other relationship; it is rewarding and fulfilling. More time with God offers a clearer perception of His direction and discernment about what He wants for you in this lifetime. Seek to spend more time with God; express love for Him with your time, energy, and attention. God loves you, and one of the best ways to love Him back is with your time.

174 | Faith over Fear in Everything

> *I sought the LORD, and he answered me;*
> *he delivered me from all my fears.*
>
> **—PSALM 34:4**

God is with us in all things; He is a present help in the time of our need. God does not leave you to face life alone. Seek God in your fearful moments. God has got you covered and will see you through anything. He has solutions to problems before they ever become problems in your life. Fear is meant to challenge you and to test your faith. Let your faith be the guiding force that wins today.

175 | Free-Flowing Grace

Out of his fullness we have all received grace in place of grace already given.

—JOHN 1:16

Grace in place of grace already given is a free-flowing grace that never changes. God perceives and understands your life experiences, and He knows the measure of grace you need to be sustained. God sustains you. He extends His grace to help you fulfill your roles and responsibilities. In the moments that feel overwhelming, remember that there is grace for the day. There is grace for your battles and for the uncertainties of life. Always remember that you have access to God's grace in life.

176 | Remaining Humble

Humble yourselves before the LORD, and he will lift you up.

—JAMES 4:10

The Bible teaches us that God exalts the humble and humbles the proud. It has often been said that if you are not humble, God will humble you. Humility is a sign of internal confidence in who God created you to be. It is a reflection of a beautiful spirit that does not seek attention, validation, and approval from people. Remaining humble when pride is tempting is an example of true strength, courage, and internal security. Your humility will bless you in life.

177 | Strength for the Weary

> *He gives strength to the weary and increases*
> *the power of the weak.*
>
> **—ISAIAH 40:29**

God strengthens you in your weary seasons. He increases your power when you feel weak. When you feel drained from constant responsibilities, remember that God can and will strengthen you. Every day that you are alive is God's way of saying that there is still so much life left for you to do, feel, experience, and enjoy. In the seasons you feel weak, ask God to provide you with supernatural strength. He provides what you need in your tough seasons. He wants to take the pressure off.

178 | Find Out What Pleases God

> *(For the fruit of the light consists in*
> *all goodness, righteousness and truth)*
> *and find out what pleases the LORD.*
>
> **—EPHESIANS 5:9–10**

What you devote your time to can either build your character and contribute to healthy living or dismantle your character and infuse negativity. The world may not always represent the heart, mind, and mission of God, but you do not have to conform to the world. Find out what pleases God. When something is not of God, it can deplete you. You are the light. Continue walking in goodness. You are deserving of a life that radiates truth, peace, love, and positivity. Prioritize godly connections.

179 | The Holy Spirit Gift

> But the Advocate, the Holy Spirit, whom the Father
> will send in my name, will teach you all things and will
> remind you of everything I have said to you.
>
> **—JOHN 14:26**

The Holy Spirit knows our heart's deepest desires. Jesus gifted us with the Holy Spirit to help us in times of need. The Holy Spirit is a friend to you. When you feel uncertain about how to speak to God, ask the Holy Spirit to help you. The Holy Spirit offers discernment, clarity, and wisdom. The Holy Spirit understands your innermost thoughts and speaks to God on your behalf. The Holy Spirit within you is powerful. The Holy Spirit offers wisdom, clarity, guidance, and comfort.

180 | When People Doubt You

> "Isn't this the carpenter? Isn't this Mary's son and the
> brother of James, Joseph, Judas and Simon? Aren't his
> sisters here with us?" And they took offense at him.
>
> **—MARK 6:3**

Sometimes what God wants to do in your life does not make sense to the people who know you or knew you in the past. Often when you begin to walk into the fullness of who God has called you to be, it will confuse people who doubted you or did not believe in the calling on your life. You will never have to prove yourself to anyone. God has already set you apart and deemed you called. Walk into your calling unapologetically.

181 | Staying Diligent

A sluggard's appetite is never filled, but the desires of the diligent are fully satisfied.

—PROVERBS 13:4

When it is hardest to work toward your dreams, remember that the greatest achievements often require diligence and sacrifice. Success is not a comfortable business, but it is one that satisfies. While it may not be comfortable to rise early or to stay up late to work toward a dream, what we work diligently for we ultimately reap satisfaction from. Dreams do not unfold without you. They need you. Always practice self-care and rest along the way, though. Rest is equally productive.

182 | Living Intentionally

Be very careful, then, how you live—not as unwise but as wise, making the most of every opportunity, because the days are evil.

—EPHESIANS 5:15–16

Paul wrote this instruction for two main reasons. First, to encourage the Ephesians to practice obedience and to carefully consider their walk with God, which is wise. Second, to remind them that life is precious. Life is only but a moment in time; live life intentionally. Make the most of every opportunity in life. The days are not ours. Though evil exists in the world, do your absolute best to lead a positive life, one that pleases God. Do your best to cultivate peace and harmony.

183 | Dismantling Dissension

> *Hatred stirs up conflict, but love covers over all wrongs.*
>
> **—PROVERBS 10:12**

Relationships require love and forgiveness. Forgiveness is not about allowing someone to keep committing the same offense, but rather deciding that your love covers their shortcoming, just as God covers yours. Hatred evokes dissension, but love births new chances. While everyone deserves forgiveness, not everyone should have a second chance at operating in the same capacity in your life. Discern wisely and lead with love: love for God, yourself, and others.

184 | A Love Like God's

> *How priceless is your unfailing love, O God! People take refuge in the shadow of your wings.*
>
> **—PSALM 36:7**

Who can find a love like God's? God's love for you is unfailing. God's love is immovable and unfaltering. His love for you is priceless. There is not a single thing that can compare or even come close to the magnitude of God's love for you. How wonderful is it to know that you can take refuge and find protection in Him? God's love for you overpowers your pains, struggles, worries, and tough seasons. His love is a strong tower and a shield of protection.

185 | The Plans in Your Heart

The heart of man plans his way, but the
LORD establishes his steps.

—PROVERBS 16:9

We may make plans in our hearts, but no plan is better than God's plan. It is normal to feel discouraged when your plans do not prevail, but when plans fail, that does not mean you will fail. Sometimes "no" means "not yet." Other times a "no" is simply God's protection. The trajectory of your life is in God's hands. God will establish your steps to align with His will because His will is perfect. God desires for His perfect will to manifest in your life.

186 | They Will Not Overcome You

"They will fight against you but will not
overcome you, for I am with you and will
rescue you," declares the LORD.

—JEREMIAH 1:19

Have you ever felt like people were against you for invalid reasons? God wants you to know that though they are against you, they will not overcome you. God will rescue you from your enemies. God will protect you from malicious attempts to attack your character and disrupt your peace. God will be your safe space in seasons where you feel alone, unsure of yourself, and rejected by mankind. God will never leave, reject, or forget you. God says you are valuable and worthy of love.

187 | God Will Comfort You

Blessed are those who mourn, for they will be comforted.

—MATTHEW 5:4

In life, we go through seasons of mourning that feel unbearable. These seasons often make us feel like the weight of the world is on our shoulders. If you have lost a loved one or have gone through a separation from someone you thought would be in your life forever, God will comfort you in this season. While He may not be able to bring that person back, He can love you and comfort you in their absence. God can overwhelm you with peace.

188 | Blessed by Obedience

Whoever heeds discipline shows the way to life, but whoever ignores correction leads others astray.

—PROVERBS 10:17

Obedience to God affects your mental health, spiritual well-being, and internal peace. God never asks us to be obedient to an instruction that we do not have the capacity to follow. God only ever requires obedience from us to protect us, safeguard us, and bless us. Being obedient to God requires discipline and self-denial. Denying ourselves simply means not succumbing to the desire to do things that are temporarily gratifying but could cause negative long-term effects. Choosing obedience blesses your life.

189 | God over Man

> *Peter and the other apostles replied: "We must obey God rather than human beings!"*
>
> **—ACTS 5:29**

While the world around us may tempt us to do things that seem societally acceptable or popular, we must remember that living for God is more important. We should not be consumed with impressing people or trying to receive their acceptance, rather we should be focused on impressing God. We cannot earn God's acceptance through obedience; we are already accepted by God, but we can choose to honor Him with our obedience. Obeying God over mankind is standing for what you believe in despite what people say.

190 | Renewed Daily

> *Therefore we do not lose heart. Though outwardly we are wasting away, yet inwardly we are being renewed day by day.*
>
> **—2 CORINTHIANS 4:16**

While we are going through life and the years are passing around us, we can find peace and contentment knowing that God renews, replenishes, and restores us internally. We are renewed day by day. That means if the grace from the day before has wasted away, God provides you with a renewed grace and peace. Not losing heart means remaining hopeful amid life's happenings. Life may be passing by, but we have access to renewed strength, mercy, and grace.

191 | Making Informed Decisions in Life

Suppose one of you wants to build a tower. Won't you first sit down and estimate the cost to see if you have enough money to complete it?

—LUKE 14:28

Jesus taught that following Him requires deep consideration of the cost. To know Christ and to follow Him is to find freedom, joy, and salvation. This parable is an example to anyone who wants to pursue a new endeavor. Calculate how the pursuit will impact your life, determine if you can fully commit, and then make the best-informed decision.

192 | Tend to Your Territory

Make it your ambition to lead a quiet life: You should mind your own business and work with your hands, just as we told you.

—1 THESSALONIANS 4:11

Paul provided the Thessalonians with life principles that are still applicable today. Making it your ambition to lead a quiet life does not mean there won't be rowdy moments; it is a reminder that living at peace with yourself and others is powerful; strive for harmony. Minding your business means tending to the territory that is yours. Minding your business minimizes the potential for conflict. Allow God to deal with people accordingly. When you focus on yourself, you improve. Work to thrive and survive.

193 | Correct Judgment

Stop judging by mere appearances,
but instead judge correctly.

—JOHN 7:24

We often find that our first impressions of people are shaped by the way they look. The true character of a person is reflected in how they treat others, though. God judges each person by their heart. God wants us to do the same. This does not mean condemning someone because of the condition of their heart; this simply means examining who they are not by how they look or by what they have but by who they are and the posture of their heart.

194 | Before Great People

A gift opens the way and ushers the giver into
the presence of the great.

—PROVERBS 18:16

Do you know that your gift makes room for you? You never have to fear that your field is oversaturated or that you cannot succeed in pursuing your dream. God will provide a space for you to thrive in your gift. God will bring you before people you admire in the field you dream of being in. God will make a way and pave a path of success for you. Your greatness will provide space for you to flourish. You are good enough to thrive.

195 | God Feels Your Pain

Jesus wept.

—JOHN 11:35

The shortest verse in the Bible is "Jesus wept." Jesus wept after seeing the pain of Lazarus dying. Jesus raised Lazarus from the dead. This verse is a reminder that God cares for the things you care about. God's heart breaks for what breaks yours. God feels your heart's pain, and He empathizes with you. God cares for you, and He is mindful of the pain you experience. He will restore your heart and bring new things to life for you. God cares for you.

196 | Be at Peace with God

My comfort in my suffering is this:
Your promise preserves my life.

—PSALM 119:50

When you are afflicted and burdened with life's challenges and difficulties, remember the promises of God. The promises of God can and will give you life. What that means is that God will comfort you and His promises will reassure you. Your situation may feel hopeless, but keep the hope. Remain hopeful that God's promises never fail. God never forgets His promises, and He is sure to deliver on His word. God will comfort you and fulfill His promises to you. God's promises will reinvigorate your hope.

197 | Trust Yourself

But blessed is the one who trusts in the LORD,
whose confidence is in him.

—JEREMIAH 17:7

Trusting God offers certainty in life. When you do not perceive what He is doing, you can have confidence in His plan for your life. Trusting God means that no matter what your life looks like right now, you can trust that God will not fail you. God believes in you; thus, you should, too. Having confidence in God could be called *God-fidence*, or the belief that because God is on your side you are destined to succeed. Things are bound to work out for your good.

198 | Search Me, Oh God

I the LORD *search the heart and examine the mind,*
to reward each person according to their
conduct, according to what their deeds deserve.

—JEREMIAH 17:10

God searches our hearts, examines our minds, and rewards each person according to their deeds. This does not mean that good works get you into Heaven; this means that God cares about the character of each person. He's concerned with seeing each person for who they are. It is a joy to know that God does not view or judge us the way others do. While others may misunderstand who we are or judge us by appearance, God examines who we are at our core.

199 | You of Little Faith

Immediately Jesus reached out his hand and caught him.
"You of little faith," he said, "why did you doubt?"

—MATTHEW 14:31

Devotion. Sometimes God wants you to do the impossible. These are supernatural moments that only God could guide you through. Peter walked on water and instantly felt like he was sinking only after he saw the wind. He allowed fear to overcome his faith. Similarly, it is not until you take your eyes and focus off of Jesus that you begin to lose sight of your power and potential. Keep your eyes on God, and He will guide you to do what others deem impossible.

200 | Calling on Jesus for Everything

The name of the LORD is a fortified tower;
the righteous run to it and are safe.

—PROVERBS 18:10

Have you ever been in a season of confusion, pain, or uncertainty? God wants you to know that His name has power. Calling on the very name of Jesus gives you power over the situations of your life. God's name is a fortified tower. That means, when you call on Jesus, His very name releases power over your life and situations. God's name provides safety, protection, love, and deliverance. Calling on God releases and activates your faith over your life. Call on Jesus for everything.

201 | God Can Rename You

> *A good name is better than fine perfume, and the day of death better than the day of birth.*
>
> **—ECCLESIASTES 7:1**

While you have no control over how others perceive you, you can always work to be the kind of person you would want to be friends with. The names that Jesus distributed were meaningful. Paul was originally Saul before his transformation and his identity as a Christian. In the same way, no past can define you. Your name can be attached to a positive reputation. God can give you a new name and a quality reputation. Being known for your identity in Christ is powerful.

202 | God Still Wants You

> *Peter replied, "Even if all fall away on account of you, I never will."*
>
> **—MATTHEW 26:33**

Peter believed that he would never fall away from Jesus. When the hour came for Jesus to be persecuted before crucifixion, Peter feared the harsh punishment he would be subjected to and went back on his word. Similarly, we may love Jesus with all of our hearts but still fall short. It is important to remember that when Jesus returned, He still desired connection and conversation with Peter. If you go back on your word to God, He still loves you and desires connection with you.

203 | Your Hope Lives On

> *There is surely a future hope for you,*
> *and your hope will not be cut off.*
>
> **—PROVERBS 23:18**

Holding on to a future hope is powerful. Do you have hope right now? What about hope for the future? There is great power in keeping your hope. While your hope may waver, keep in mind that hope is confidence in God. God will make a new way for you to prevail. God will heal and deliver you. God will align you with the right people and connections. God will give you hope for future blessings, and this hope will not be deferred.

204 | His Love Endures Forever

> *The LORD will vindicate me; your love, LORD, endures*
> *forever—do not abandon the works of your hands.*
>
> **—PSALM 138:8**

The Lord will vindicate you. He loves you; His love for you endures forever. Not abandoning the works of your hands means that God will bring to completion all of the good works that He began in you. God remembers you in all things and keeps you protected and under the wing of His mighty care and love. He will ensure that the gifts He put in you manifest the fruit of your labor. He will establish you and set you apart for greatness.

205 | Be Mindful of Your Company

> *Do not make friends with a hot-tempered person, do not associate with one easily angered, or you may learn their ways and get yourself ensnared.*
>
> **—PROVERBS 22:24–25**

It is vital that you are mindful of the impact poor company has on you. While we cannot control when someone we love has a bad temper, we can practice caution so as to avoid dynamics with people whose temper is reflected in every tough situation. What you allow yourself to be around consistently can eventually show up in your character. The more you associate with angry people, the angrier you can become. The company you keep can be the reward or the detriment you reap.

206 | God Never Changes

> *I the LORD do not change. So you, the descendants of Jacob, are not destroyed.*
>
> **—MALACHI 3:6**

This was a reminder to the Israelites that their survival was a result of God's faithfulness and promises. In the same way, your existence is a result of God's consistency, love, grace, and mercy. God's perfect promises to you and his faithfulness are sustenance to you. God's unchanging character is why you are sustained and kept in His heart. While mankind may waver in love, character, and commitment, God remains the same.

207 | Wholesome Talk

> *Those who consider themselves religious and yet do not keep a tight rein on their tongues deceive themselves, and their religion is worthless.*
>
> **—JAMES 1:26**

Identifying with Christ means working to have self-control in our speech; it means keeping oneself from slanderous talk. It can be tempting to join in on gossip, but gossip causes division and dissension, which is in direct opposition to what God would have for His children. Gossip can reveal the most unattractive thoughts we have toward someone. Strive to see the best in people, and when you can't, avoid speaking ill of people. Our words can either be a light or a dark pit.

208 | Spreading the Good News

> *He said to them, "Go into all the world and preach the gospel to all creation."*
>
> **—MARK 16:15**

No matter what your gift is, there is a great chance that you can spread the good news using it. Your gift can be used to serve the Kingdom of God and to share the good news. The disciples were unlearned and had varying backgrounds, yet each used their lives to testify about Jesus. In the same way, you may encounter people who do not know Jesus. Be unashamed of the Gospel and share the good news. Your obedience may be what saves someone.

209 | Ability to Apologize

> *Whoever conceals their sins does not prosper, but the one who confesses and renounces them finds mercy.*
>
> **—PROVERBS 28:13**

This verse is a reminder that God is faithful in forgiving us our sins, though something to consider is confessing our wrongdoings to the people we've wronged. We must be willing to take ownership for our actions when they are wrong and apologize when needed. We must understand that God wants us to be honest with ourselves and others. The ability to be unified with others stems from our willingness to be loving, kind, and forgiving but to also extend apologies when needed.

210 | The Value of Persisting

> *But as for you, be strong and do not give up, for your work will be rewarded.*
>
> **—2 CHRONICLES 15:7**

Do you ever feel like giving up and letting go? Understand that God does not give up on your dream and He does not want you to give up, either. Rest along the way, grant yourself breaks, and practice self-care, but persist. Understand that God bestows strength unto each person who needs it. If you keep pressing on and keep refusing to give up, your work will reward you. What you work for will produce favorable results. Keep working and watch your labor produce blessings.

211 | Be Bold and Assertive

Therefore, since we have such a hope, we are very bold.

—2 CORINTHIANS 3:12

Christians can be confident in who they are because of their association with a perfect King. Being coheirs with Christ means you have the capacity to be bold and assertive. This does not mean to forsake humility, but rather to be confident and unashamed of who you are and what you believe in as a Christian. You have the capacity to speak boldly and authoritatively. You deserve to be heard and seen. You deserve to unapologetically take up space. You are a Child of the King.

212 | The Best Version of You

As obedient children, do not conform to the evil desires you had when you lived in ignorance.

—1 PETER 1:14

It is easy to revert to old habits, even though being a Christian means we vowed to forsake old patterns that were not conducive to our new identity in Christ. We won't be perfect, but we can grow. Work to improve yourself. Being a Christian means working to be the best version of yourself. While you may backslide, pick yourself up and start again. Eventually, who you desire to become will emerge and take up space in an unapologetic way. She will be immovable and unshakable.

213 | Creating New Habits

> *Follow God's example, therefore, as dearly loved children.*
>
> **—EPHESIANS 5:1**

While we won't be perfect like God, we can work to keep our hearts, minds, and actions aligned with His. When we study the life of Jesus, in how He carried Himself and treated others, we see how we should conduct ourselves. We can create habits that align with His character. We can practice speaking kindly to others and loving them unconditionally. We can designate time for prayer and cultivate healthy friendships. When we follow God's example, we see positive impacts in our lives.

214 | Holy Spirit Gifts

> *There are different kinds of service, but the same* LORD.
>
> **—1 CORINTHIANS 12:5**

The Holy Spirit gifts each person differently. No one gift deems one person more important than the next. God values all of His children the same. Each gift is given for glorifying God. If you ever feel tempted to compare your gifts, the level of your gifts, or the lack of gifts to someone else's, be reminded that gifts do not make a person more or less valuable, spiritual, or important. Each being is spiritual. The gifts are simply bestowed according to the Holy Spirit's discretion.

215 | The Lord's Compassion

The LORD is compassionate and gracious,
slow to anger, abounding in love.

—PSALM 103:8

What a joy it is to know that God is compassionate, gracious, slow to anger, and abounding in love. God is not like man, who may lack compassion for you when you need it most. God is not unforgiving, like some people have been toward you. God is not easily angered, like some humans you know are. God loves you unconditionally. His love is not confined or based on actions you perform. God's love is not predicated on how much you do right.

216 | Set an Example

Don't let anyone look down on you because you are
young, but set an example for the believers in speech,
in conduct, in love, in faith and in purity.

—1 TIMOTHY 4:12

If God calls you to something, people do not have to understand it for you to be effective in that calling. Do not allow people to belittle how powerful and valuable you are. Wherever you are, set an example and continue to be the light. You may encounter jealous naysayers who attempt to minimize your gifts and talents, but you only need validation from God. Once God has deemed you worthy, you are capable, whether others agree with that truth or not.

217 | Jesus Provides Spiritual Sustenance

Then Jesus declared, "I am the bread of life.
Whoever comes to me will never go hungry, and
whoever believes in me will never be thirsty."

—JOHN 6:35

Many people look to fill their spiritual appetites with things that will not give them true fulfillment, internal content-ment, and joy. Being reliant on Jesus fills and fuels you. Having a relationship with Jesus fills your spiritual tank and causes you to overflow with peace, love, joy, harmony, and abundance. The truth is that nothing and no one can fill us up the way Jesus can. When we begin to rely on that truth, we see our lives changing and enhancing for the better.

218 | Allow God to Refresh You

I will refresh the weary and satisfy the faint.

—JEREMIAH 31:25

Feeling drained and exhausted? God will refresh you. God will provide you with stamina for the journey. God replen-ishes your endurance and gives you supernatural strength for the journey. Obstacles may surface, but God wants you to be fit for the journey so that you can walk into the abun-dance of blessings that comes with persisting. God always prepares you for the journey of your life. He desires to see the things you pursue in this life come to completion. He desires to see you through tough seasons.

219 | Following Jesus and Self-Denial

> Then Jesus said to his disciples, "Whoever wants
> to be my disciple must deny themselves and take up
> their cross and follow me."
>
> **—MATTHEW 16:24**

Following Jesus is an act of self-denial. While this is not always easy, it is always worth the sacrifice. God's sacrifice for mankind was supernatural love. If all He asks for in return is to follow Him and to deny fleshly desires, then we can do our best to do that. God simply wants our hearts and our minds. He wants us to be committed to following Him and to cast down any behaviors and relationships that threaten our commitment to Him. You are free in Him.

220 | Empathy and Compassion Like Jesus

> Rejoice with those who rejoice;
> mourn with those who mourn.
>
> **—ROMANS 12:15**

Empathy and compassion are characteristics of Jesus. Christ was supremely empathetic and compassionate toward strangers, though. In the same way, being Christ-like means reflecting a heart of compassion for others. We may not perceive other people's experiences or grasp the severity of how they have been impacted adversely, but we can empathize and show up for them in a valuable way. We can model God's love.

221 | God's Infinite Power

> *Ah, Sovereign LORD, you have made the heavens and the earth by your great power and outstretched arm. Nothing is too hard for you.*
>
> **—JEREMIAH 32:17**

Do you perceive how powerful God is? There is nothing too hard for God. He is not limited or confined. God is all knowing and all powerful. He has the power to do what no man can. God is not intimidated by the giants of your life. God does not fear the tough things that surface. God is all powerful. He has the power to show up at any moment in time and create a solution for your need. God created and controls the universe.

222 | Jesus the Healer

> *He said to her, "Daughter, your faith has healed you. Go in peace and be freed from your suffering."*
>
> **—MARK 5:34**

God can heal you from any infirmity; faith in God is all you need. A woman was hemorrhaging for 12 years, but she had faith that if she touched the hem of the garment Jesus was wearing she would be healed. She was instantly healed. Jesus told her that it was her faith that healed her. Have faith that God can and will heal you despite the severity of the diagnosis and the amount of time you have been fighting for healing.

223 | Praise God with Dancing

Let them praise his name with dancing and make music to him with timbrel and harp.

—PSALM 149:3

Do you know that you can dance unto the Lord in worship? Dancing for God can free you from the weight of life stressors. Praise God through dance and music today. Let Him know how much you love to worship and praise Him. Your praise never gets old to God. He loves to see you celebrate your love for Him. Worship does not have to be confined to one particular method. You can dance like David danced and worship the Lord with music.

224 | God Is Your Help

Surely God is my help; the LORD is the one who sustains me.

—PSALM 54:4

Have you ever felt like no one knew how to help you? Maybe you have even felt like no one knew you needed help. Whatever the case, God is your help. God can help you through anything. God does not hold it against you or expect any favors in return when you ask for help. God helps you because He loves you. He wants to sustain and deliver you. He wants your needs to be met. God is a faithful friend and a loyal companion.

225 | Your Gifts

> *They saw what seemed to be tongues of fire that separated and came to rest on each of them.*
>
> **—ACTS 2:3**

The disciples received the gifts of tongues. While you may not have had this experience in your walk with Christ, you have gifts that testify to the power of God. Do you know what your supernatural gifts are? Each gift granted you is an identifier of the God who created you. God wanted the world to see Him reflected in you. Whatever your gifts are, use them with a gracious awareness of where it came from. Your gifts are God's way of loving people through you.

226 | God Is Always Faithful

> *For the word of the LORD is right and true; he is faithful in all he does.*
>
> **—PSALM 33:4**

Whenever you do not know what to think, believe, or feel, read the Word of God. There are some certainties and absolutes and a few of them are that God never changes, His Word never comes back void, false, or inaccurate, and He loves you unconditionally. It does not matter what chaos ensues in your life, there is always a faithful King whose Words will always be right and true. You can rely on Him in every season of your life. You can always trust God.

227 | The Armor of God

> *Rather, clothe yourselves with the* LORD
> *Jesus Christ, and do not think about how to*
> *gratify the desires of the flesh.*
>
> **—ROMANS 13:14**

To put on the Armor of God and to clothe yourself with
Jesus Christ means to protect yourself from wrongdoing.
It also means to guard yourself from going into the world
spiritually naked. Out in the world, we encounter things
that can be disruptive and toxic to our walk with Christ.
Clothing yourself with Jesus simply means arming yourself with His Word and spending time in prayer. When you
clothe yourself with Jesus, you are less likely to succumb to
worldly temptation.

228 | Highly Favored

> *For God does not show favoritism.*
>
> **—ROMANS 2:11**

God does not show favoritism, but He does favor His children. Genesis 6:8 tells us that Noah found favor with the
Lord. What we need to remember is that being a Child of
God sets us apart. It does not make us better than anyone
else, it simply means we are saved. We are redeemed,
restored, and made new in Christ. We are His children. We
do not belong to the world. We act according to His Word
and follow His direction for our lives.

229 | An On-Time God

> *Sarah became pregnant and bore a son to Abraham in his old age, at the very time God had promised him.*
>
> **—GENESIS 21:2**

It is never too late to experience the goodness of God. If you have been waiting for a promise from God, remember that God is never late. We serve an on-time God who remembers the timing of His promises. God knew that Abraham and Sarah would live long lives, so He fulfilled His promise to them in their old age because the timing of their lives was in His hands. Likewise, the timing of your life is in God's hands. God never runs out of time.

230 | A House Built on Rock

> *Therefore everyone who hears these words of mine and puts them into practice is like a wise man who built his house on the rock.*
>
> **—MATTHEW 7:24**

A house built on the rock is a house built to last. This house can withstand any storm, inclement weather, or attack. Understand that your faith grounds you. Your faith in God safeguards you from crippling and destructive attacks. Anyone who lives their life according to the Word lives their life wisely. When you are rooted in God, He takes root in you. Being rooted in God provides you safety from the world. Being rooted in God gives you a first-class ticket to Heaven.

231 | Established Plans

> *Commit to the* LORD *whatever you do, and he will establish your plans.*
>
> **—PROVERBS 16:3**

When you commit to God in all that you do, He aligns your path with His plan for your life. The best path to be on is one of divine orchestration and manifestation. When you commit to the Lord, He ensures that the right doors of opportunities open, and the appropriate connections are made. God ensures your success. Seamless experiences are a reflection of God's divine orchestration at work in your life. Your commitment to His plan for your life will bless you effortlessly.

232 | Open Mind for Scripture

> *Then he opened their minds so they could understand the Scriptures.*
>
> **—LUKE 24:45**

Jesus often spoke in parables because people struggled to understand Him. In the same way, we live in a time where reading the Bible is not habitual. How can we learn, grow, and connect with God intimately if we never delve into the love letter that is the Bible? The beautiful thing is that if we dedicate time to learning what the Word of God says, we can ask Him to open our minds to help us understand and receive the messages being relayed.

233 | Justified through Faith

For it is with your heart that you believe and are justified, and it is with your mouth that you profess your faith and are saved.

—ROMANS 10:10

Your faith justifies you. When your heart reflects love and acceptance for Jesus and your mouth confesses that He is your savior, you are sealed. Our heart's posture and our mouth's admittance to Jesus are declarative factors of our identity in Christ. You are not justified by good behavior, sinless deeds, and a likable personality; you are justified by your faith in Jesus Christ. God examines our hearts. Our hearts are a reflection of who we are and who we stand for. Stand tall for Jesus.

234 | Seize Each New Day

Teach us to number our days, that we may gain a heart of wisdom.

—PSALM 90:12

The days are not ours. Time belongs to God. Moses prayed that God would give him the ability to see each new day as one to cherish rather than one to squander. Work to dismantle whatever has been wasting your time or delaying your destiny. The days are precious, short, and valuable. Keep God at the center of each day. Strive to be at peace with yourself and others. Be obedient to the Word of God and practice wisdom in all that you commit yourself to.

235 | You Overcome

> *For everyone born of God overcomes the world. This is the victory that has overcome the world, even our faith.*
>
> **—1 JOHN 5:4**

As a child of God, nothing in the world can overcome you. Weapons may form, but they will not prosper. Naysayers may open their mouths against you, but their words will fail. Problems and battles may be heavy, but God defends you. God brings about solutions before problems begin to form. You are the child of an undebatable King who sits high, looks low, and is mindful of you in all things. God will not let any harm overcome you. He protects and covers you.

236 | Humility, Riches, and Honor

> *Humility is the fear of the LORD; its wages are riches and honor and life.*
>
> **—PROVERBS 22:4**

Being a humble servant of the Lord provides for a fruitful and honorable life. While there are blessings on Earth, nothing amounts to the blessings in Heaven. Heaven houses an abundance of blessings for the humble in spirit. God designed us to humbly love others. A life that reflects humility is honorable to God. Riches are not always materialistic and monetary. In fact, some of the greatest riches are good health, strong family dynamics, peace, love, and harmony. Choose humility and reap riches and honor.

237 | Hardship Produces Perseverance

Not only so, but we also glory in our sufferings, because we know that suffering produces perseverance.

—ROMANS 5:3

Paul stated that our sufferings produce perseverance. Additionally, sometimes seasons of hardship draw us closer to God. Whenever we feel like no one else understands or there isn't anything anyone can do, we are compelled to rely on God. Some seasons draw us to our knees because that is the best place to be. Those seasons require our humility, prayer, and total reliance on God. Thus, to glory or rejoice in suffering means to relish in the belief that God will eventually see you through.

238 | Holy Spirit Power in You

Now Stephen, a man full of God's grace and power, performed great wonders and signs among the people.

—ACTS 6:8

The Holy Spirit gave Stephen grace and power. Additionally, Stephen was able to perform wonders and signs. Despite who he was and all that he could do, people found a way to argue and attack him. But according to the Bible, despite their dislike for Stephen, they could not deny the wisdom the Spirit gave him. This is an indicator that there will be some people committed to disliking you, but despite their dislike, they will have no choice but to respect the Holy Spirit's work in you.

239 | Salvation for Everyone

> *For the grace of God has appeared that*
> *offers salvation to all people.*
>
> **—TITUS 2:11**

Salvation is for everyone. God loves and wants relationships with everyone. He is deeply loving and forgiving. He simply wants His children to come to Him and to be saved. Salvation was not only for the most well-behaved people on Earth; in fact, Jesus came for the sick—the sick in spirit, mind, body, and soul. He came because He knew we needed a redeemer. Seek to speak to those who feel like they are out of God's reach. Let them know that salvation is for them.

240 | Increase My Faith, Lord

> *The apostles said to the LORD, "Increase our faith!"*
>
> **—LUKE 17:5**

Ask God to increase your faith. God says all you need is faith the size of a mustard seed. A mustard seed is tiny! Ask God to give you wild faith. Faith is vital to your hope. It keeps you believing in what you are waiting for. When you need a breakthrough, ask God to increase your faith so that it matches the magnitude of the blessings coming your way. What you have the capacity to believe in, God has the capacity to manifest, and He's a multiplier.

241 | You Are Holy and Blameless

For he chose us in him before the creation of the world to be holy and blameless in his sight.

—EPHESIANS 1:4

How powerful is it to know that God chose you before He created the world? Do you perceive that He created the universe and everything in it and then created mankind? He saved the best for last. God has always known you. He has known you before you were formed in your mother's womb. He has always chosen you, set you apart, and loved you. To be holy means to walk differently because you are His. God views you as a divine manifestation of His love.

242 | Anchor Yourself in Faith

Resist him, standing firm in the faith, because you know that the family of believers throughout the world is undergoing the same kind of sufferings.

—1 PETER 5:9

Anchor yourself in your faith. When you anchor yourself in faith, it gives you strength, resilience, persistence, and hope. Standing firm in your faith is vital to fighting the battles of your life. What may offer you consolation is knowing that you are never alone. If you join with fellow believers, you will find that everyone undergoes struggles and fellow Christians often experience similar struggles. You might find many commonalities in your story and that of your Christian friends. Your testimony can inspire faith in others.

243 | Declare His Name

*I will declare your name to my people; in the
assembly I will praise you.*

—PSALM 22:22

David praised God and declared His name because God
gave David victory over his enemies. Similarly, you will have
victory over your enemies. There will come a time when the
people who thought they had a final say over your life will
see God's hand in your life. The battles and the enemies of
your life are still under God's direction and authority. It may
appear as if your enemies are getting away with mistreating
you, but God sees all and He will vindicate you.

244 | Bring the Dark to Light

*Have nothing to do with the fruitless deeds of
darkness, but rather expose them.*

—EPHESIANS 5:11

Have nothing to do with fruitless deeds. Do not dabble or
wallow in sinful behaviors and habits. What you spend your
time doing will affect your life. Sinful behaviors will not
provide for a fruitful life. When you expose anything, you call
it out, name it what it is, and get direct about how it affects
your life. Paul instructs believers to steer clear of fruitless
deeds and expose them. When you stay away from sin and
expose sin, you walk in light and truth.

245 | Invite Others In

For many are invited, but few are chosen.

—MATTHEW 22:14

God chooses His children, but not everyone chooses Him back. God desires for everyone to experience Heaven. The invitation to Heaven is a result of accepting His initial invitation to be in a relationship with Him. While you may have already accepted the invitation to a relationship with God, it is important to share with others how valuable they are to God. Some people only experience God through Christians. Be the Christian that tells people that God is inviting them into a relationship with Him.

246 | You Are a Necessary Creation

For you created my inmost being; you knit me together in my mother's womb.

—PSALM 139:13

God has created you specifically for a divine purpose. God is an artist, and He created you intricately. He knows you intimately and loves you deeply. He created all of your quirks, tendencies, skills, and talents. He knit you in your mother's womb. You were designed by the Creator of the Universe, made for a divine purpose and destined for greatness. The Artist of All Artists created you. He deemed you a necessary creation of His perfect design.

247 | Love God, Love Others

And he has given us this command: Anyone who loves God must also love their brother and sister.

—1 JOHN 4:21

Most people would agree that it is not easy to love every single person in the world, but God does call us to love Him and to love others. Loving others, particularly when they are not being easy to love, is an ultimate reflection of God. The best way to radiate God's love is to love. While not everyone is easy to love, God never called us to decipher between who is deserving of love and who is not. Loving God means loving others.

248 | A Wise Woman

The wise woman builds her house, but with her own hands the foolish one tears hers down.

—PROVERBS 14:1

Solomon was describing how valuable women are and how much of an asset they are to their homes. A house built on faith and wisdom contributes to the healthy ebb and flow of a woman's home. Neglecting your faith, relationship with God, or forsaking the needs of yourself and family can cause disruption in your home. While women often have a great deal to manage at once, always remember to value your relationship with God above all else and to keep unshakable faith.

249 | Wisdom from God over Mankind

> This is what the LORD says: "Cursed is the one who trusts in man, who draws strength from mere flesh and whose heart turns away from the LORD."
>
> **—JEREMIAH 17:5**

At one point or another, we have all relied on our people for guidance about our life. This verse comes from a time when people relied on humans more than God. God is the ultimate source of guidance, strength, and wisdom. A heart and mind rooted in God is wise. Our trust and faith should be in God above all else. God always has the final say. Rather than relying more on the wisdom of mankind, we should seek guidance from God.

250 | Trust in the Lord in All Things

> Whoever gives heed to instruction prospers, and blessed is the one who trusts in the LORD.
>
> **—PROVERBS 16:20**

It may be difficult to receive constructive feedback, but it is wise to apply feedback that could potentially catapult your ventures in life. No one knows everything except for God. The person who relies chiefly on their own knowledge, expertise, and wisdom shortchanges themselves. Trusting in the Lord and depending on His guidance offers a certainty about prospering in professional pursuits in life.

251 | Honest Gain Lasts a Lifetime

> *Such are the paths of all who go after ill-gotten gain;*
> *it takes away the life of those who get it.*
>
> **—PROVERBS 1:19**

Watching people flourish who have hurt others to get what they have can be painful. Remember that God knows everything. Things that are ill-gotten do not last. If it defies God's design for peace, harmony, and honesty, it will not prevail. Always be proud of your honest gain through pure intentions. It does not matter how successful one may appear, if they have done wrong to be where they are, what they have will not last. What you work for honestly will bless you.

252 | The Little Moments

> *But the LORD answered and said to her, "Martha, Martha,*
> *you are worried and bothered about so many things."*
>
> **—LUKE 10:41**

Jesus kindly told Martha that she does not have to worry herself with preparations and duties to provide Jesus with a pleasant time. Jesus wanted Martha to enjoy that moment in time with Him. Similarly, we may busy ourselves with a clean home or perfect preparation and miss quality moments that could be best spent enjoying family. Time is fleeting, and moments with loved ones are not promised. Thus, it is valuable to put tasks away sometimes and simply embrace the presence of loved ones.

253 | Divine Orchestration

> For the LORD Almighty has purposed, and
> who can thwart him? His hand is stretched out,
> and who can turn it back?
>
> **—ISAIAH 14:27**

God is all powerful and undefeatable. Your situation may
look hopeless, people may not believe in you, and the
cards may seem stacked against you, but what God has in
store for you will prevail against all odds. The thing about
divine orchestration is that its place does not waver, and its
plans unfold no matter what. God cannot be stopped. What
God has purposed for your life cannot be thwarted. When
His hand is over your life, there is nothing that can inhibit
what He has for you.

254 | The Power of God's Word

> The unfolding of Your words gives light; it gives
> understanding to the simple.
>
> **—PSALM 119:130**

God is the Creator and Originator of Language. God so
desired communication with mankind that He created language. His Words give light; His Words give understanding and
wisdom. When you are uncertain of things, when you simply
need direction or insight, read the Word of God. God's Word
offers hope, direction, and clarity. Meditating on God's Word
consistently is valuable to your inner life. Meditating on the
Word of God contributes to inner peace, confidence, and
tranquility. His Word offers comfort and assurance.

255 | Faith Walk

As the body without the spirit is dead, so faith without deeds is dead.

—JAMES 2:26

Have active faith. Faith is taking steps without seeing the entire staircase. Faith is trusting that God will catch you when you take big leaps. Taking leaps of faith may feel risky, but the greater risk lies in never acting on your faith. When we act on our faith, it shows God that we trust Him. Acting on your faith shows God that you believe in Him, His supernaturality, and His plan. Work to have active faith. Do things that support your faith walk.

256 | Self-Control

Like a city whose walls are broken through is a person who lacks self-control.

—PROVERBS 25:28

Self-control is not the easiest feat, but it protects against things not meant for you. Self-control is protection from overindulgence, wrong choices, and unfavorable outcomes. When we think about a city whose walls are broken, we must consider how unsafe and exposed broken walls are. Without self-control, we are exposed to the possibility of making decisions that can affect us poorly for a lifetime. Discernment is wisdom offered by the Holy Spirit; strive to use discernment and practice self-control.

257 | Overlooking Insults

> *Fools show their annoyance at once, but the prudent overlook an insult.*
>
> **—PROVERBS 12:16**

Being easily vexed and irritated causes tension in your interactions. Rather than becoming defensive or offended, overlook insults and keep your peace. It is harmful when we allow someone else's poor treatment, poor choice of words, or offensive behaviors to dictate our life experiences. People should never have enough power over your life that it determines your level of peace and joy for the day. If you find that someone consistently challenges your peace, set boundaries, create space, or reframe how you receive the person.

258 | No Pain Measures Up

> *I consider that our present sufferings are not worth comparing with the glory that will be revealed in us.*
>
> **—ROMANS 8:18**

No matter what pains arise in your life, the God of the universe says those pains do not compare to the glory that is to be revealed in you. This means you may have come from a broken home, an abusive childhood or marriage, or a toxic relationship, but God says the magnitude of your problems and pains do not compare to the joy that is to come. The pains of your past do not compare to all that God will do through you and for you.

259 | He Who Is without Sin

*When they kept on questioning him, he straightened
up and said to them, "Let any one of you who is without
sin be the first to throw a stone at her."*

—JOHN 8:7

Jesus had compassion for a woman accused of adultery.
Her critics surrounded her and questioned Jesus about
stoning her for her sin. Jesus knew this woman was being
judged harshly. He explained to her critics that no one is
without sin. In the same way, when people try to label you
by your mistakes, remind them who your God is. Your God
is loving and forgiving. God does not see you through the
same lens that mankind does. God deems you forgiven,
loved, whole, and worthy.

260 | Saved and Knowledgeable

*This is good, and pleases our Savior,
who wants all people to be saved and to
come to a knowledge of the truth.*

—1 TIMOTHY 2:3–4

God wants everyone to be saved and come to the knowledge
of truth. You may encounter people with different belief
systems or even have family and friends who have different
beliefs about God. The most powerful thing you can do is
be the example God calls you to be. You do not have to be
an overbearing Christian; you can simply keep praying for
them. Work to navigate conversations with grace and compassion. When you plant the seed of knowledge, God brings
it to fruition.

261 | Go Where You Are Wanted

*If anyone will not welcome you or listen to your words,
leave that home or town and shake the dust off your feet.*

—MATTHEW 10:14

Jesus told the apostles to teach that the Kingdom of Heaven is near. As He sent the apostles off, He instructed them not to dwell in spaces where they were not received and accepted. Jesus taught them to do their part but not to feel culpable for those who do not appreciate what they teach. Similarly, do not allow other people's rejection of you to deter you from your mission. Protect yourself from spaces with people who are unaccepting and intolerant of you and your mission.

262 | Do Good Unto Others

*And do not forget to do good and to share with others,
for with such sacrifices God is pleased.*

—HEBREWS 13:16

You know who needs your talents, gifts, and abilities? The world. You have a tremendous amount to offer the world. Your uniqueness is valuable. You are one of a kind. What is inside of you matters. How you create and perform is necessary. You may view your gifts as ordinary, but they are invaluable and beautiful. Your gifts are not useless; use your gifts to glorify God, to honor His Word, and to bless others. What you do to serve others pleases God.

263 | Love Your Neighbor as Yourself

Do not seek revenge or bear a grudge against anyone among your people, but love your neighbor as yourself. I am the LORD.

—LEVITICUS 19:18

Sometimes when we are deeply offended, we are tempted to hold a grudge and seek revenge. Holding grudges is toxic to your internal well-being. You do not deserve to carry the heaviness of someone else's mistakes and poor treatment. Grudges are heavy burdens that disrupt your peace. It may feel like seeking revenge will even the score, but the truth is that human revenge never settles your spirit. Allow God to issue consequences accordingly. Work to love them despite their offense toward you.

264 | Accountability

So then, each of us will give an account of ourselves to God.

—ROMANS 14:12

Accountability is self-awareness and ownership of your behaviors, habits, and interactions. When you meet God, you will not give an account of anyone else but yourself. You will tell God who you were and what you did in this lifetime. What will be your story? What are you doing in your life today that makes God proud? This verse is not to scare believers but to call them to attention. Water your grass and focus on being the best person you can be.

265 | Grace

Gracious words are a honeycomb, sweet to the soul and healing to the bones.

—PROVERBS 16:24

Gracious words free people. The world is filled with harsh words, negative remarks, and unfavorable encounters, but a gracious word offers the soul healing. We need more grace, peace, and kindness in the world. We cannot teach everyone grace, but we can model it for everyone we encounter. We can be the grace someone needed. Grace offers healing because it is not found everywhere. When Jesus walked this Earth, He exuded grace. In the same way, we should show people God's grace—that is, loving thy neighbor.

266 | Love

Dear children, let us not love with words or speech but with actions and in truth.

—1 JOHN 3:18

Love is actionable. When we truly love God, ourselves, and others, it shows in our actions. Authentic love is reflected in how we do things and in how we treat others. Love is not just a confession of our sentiments toward someone, love is behavior, outward declarations, and gestures. Love is seen in how we speak to someone and about them. Love is modeled in the things we do for someone and the things we avoid because we love them. Love is genuine actions and intentions.

267 | Glorify God

> *Because your love is better than life,*
> *my lips will glorify you.*
>
> **—PSALM 63:3**

God's love is better than life. His love sustains you in tough seasons, delivers you, and restores your health. God's love is what opens doors for you and aligns the right connections. God's love causes your doubters to be fooled and your enemies to see your blessings. God's love makes the impossible possible. God's love covers your sins, wakes you up in the morning, and encamps angels around you. God's love redeems you, surrounds you, and protects you. Glorify God; His love is better than life.

268 | Victory over Your Life

> *When the angel of the LORD appeared to Gideon, he said,*
> *"The LORD is with you, mighty warrior."*
>
> **—JUDGES 6:12**

When God deems you a mighty warrior, He is declaring victory over your life. God is your teammate because He wants you to be a mighty warrior in life. He wants you to defeat the battles and enemies of your life. A warrior is a brave fighter. Bravely combat those things that seek to take your peace. Maybe for you the battle is within. Whatever the battle is, God wants you to have victory. Victory over sadness, anxiety, depression, uncertainty, doubt, and anger.

269 | Be a Blessing, See Blessings

At this they wept aloud again. Then Orpah kissed her mother-in-law goodbye, but Ruth clung to her.

—RUTH 1:14

There is value in loyalty and commitment. Naomi lost her husband and her sons, so she instructed her daughters-in-law to move on with their lives. Ruth refuses to leave her mother-in-law; Ruth vows to stay and care for her. Ruth's loyalty gave her the opportunity to remarry into wealth and to care for Naomi. Ruth was not looking for a blessing; she became one and then received one. Becoming a blessing to someone else can provide you with unexpected blessings.

270 | Stay with God and Strengthen

And David became more and more powerful, because the LORD God of Heaven's Armies were with him.

—2 SAMUEL 5:10

God protects, covers, and favors you. David was a mighty warrior in battle, a king, and a leader. He was not without sin, though; despite his shortcomings, God favored him. David's increasing strength and power is attributed to God being with Him. You are equipped, qualified, strengthened, and capable of fulfilling the calling and mission of your life. The Lord will strengthen and empower you because He is with you. Keeping God with you provides you with renewed strength and continual growth; ultimately, you prevail.

271 | A Faithful and Providing God

The LORD heard Elijah's cry, and the boy's life returned to him, and he lived.

—1 KING 17:22

Elijah stayed with a poor widow and her son while God provided for them. Suddenly, the widow's son fell ill and died. Elijah took her son and cried out to God to restore his life. When God heard Elijah's cry, the boy's life returned to him. This story reveals a few things about God's character. God will provide for you. He will send people to love and care for you. God can revive and restore a dead and hopeless situation. God cares about your heart's cry.

272 | Fire from God

Then the fire of the LORD fell and burned up the sacrifice, the wood, the stones and the soil, and also licked up the water in the trench.

—1 KINGS 18:38

Elijah instructed Baal worshippers to choose their god. In a display of which god had real power and authority, the people called on Baal, though nothing happened. Elijah called on God, and God sent fire from Heaven. Be cautious not to make anything outside of God, your God. Humans have a tendency to value things, people, and places more than God. Analyze who is getting the best of you. Ensure that nothing is taking the place of God in your life.

273 | God Is Serious about You

> *Do not touch my anointed ones; do my prophets no harm.*
>
> **—PSALM 105:15**

God is serious about His children. He does not take mistreatment of His children lightly. It is comforting to know that God protects, defends, and avenges us. No matter what anyone on this Earth does to you or against you, God will not only protect you, but He will defend you against them. No matter what anyone says against you, the truth about you is found in God's Word. You never have to stand alone against your enemies; God will always stand with you.

274 | Your Work Will Be Rewarded

> *But as for you, be strong and do not give up, for your work will be rewarded.*
>
> **—2 CHRONICLES 15:7**

You may not get recognition from man. You may not get acknowledgment from your boss or family and friends, but your hard work is never in vain. God acknowledges you and sees your efforts. God knows how hard you work. God recognizes how much effort you put into making your dreams come true. He sees your late nights and early mornings. Keep standing strong in your gifts and calling. Keep pushing and pursuing more for yourself. In due season, your work will be rewarded.

275 | Prioritize Your Calling

Four times they sent me the same message, and each time I gave the same reply.

—NEHEMIAH 6:4

There were people attempting to harm Nehemiah and inhibit his progress. Nehemiah was committed to his calling and denied their request to meet him. Sometimes people envy your work; these people do not support you and may mean harm. Unapologetically commit to your mission to fulfill the call of God in your life. Set boundaries and cultivate unwavering standards for people in your space. Do not let people dissuade you from fulfilling your mission. Do not allow people to distract you from your calling.

276 | Your Sacrifices Will Go Far

Esther had not revealed her nationality and family background, because Mordecai had forbidden her to do so.

—ESTHER 2:10

Esther sacrificed a great deal to protect her people and her family. When we sacrifice for others, God honors the sacrifice. God will position you, favor you, promote you, and align you with the right people to assist you in making a difference in your community and in your family. Your sacrifices will bless generations to come. Your commitment will catapult you and those you love. What you vow to do and the work you commit to ultimately bless you and the generations to come.

277 | Trust Him Anyway

Though he slay me, yet will I hope in him; I will surely defend my ways to his face.

—JOB 13:15

Job did not understand why he was experiencing a great deal of hardship, but Job vowed to trust God and to remain hopeful. Job never blamed God. God placed stipulations on how far Job's affliction could be taken. Similarly, no matter what transpires in your life, God is still good. Though you struggle, keep your hope and trust in Him. He will keep you. God will not let you be consumed in the fire of your life's struggles. Like Job, in tough seasons, trust God anyway.

278 | No More Little Foxes

Catch for us the foxes, the little foxes that ruin the vineyards, our vineyards that are in bloom.

—SONG OF SONGS 2:15

Catching the little foxes has to do with nipping things in the bud. Not allowing distractions and nonhelpful habits to take up space in your life. Catching the little foxes is about paying attention to what is ruining your work and inhibiting your progression. If you want to progress and do well, then you must be intentional about eliminating what does not belong in your space. Sometimes that means cutting ties with people, places, and old habits. You can do what needs to be done to flourish.

279 | Endless Love and Mercy

> *Because of the* Lord's *great love we are not consumed,*
> *for his compassions never fail. They are*
> *new every morning; great is your faithfulness.*
>
> **—LAMENTATIONS 3:22-23**

God's love, mercy, and compassion for you never fails. His mercy is made new every morning. The Lord's love for you is never consumed. God has genuine compassion for you. Even when you feel like you are undeserving of grace, God still has compassion for you. God's mercy is new every morning because He knows we need new grace for each day. He is truly a faithful God, who deserves all of the praise, honor, and glory.

280 | Tell of His Miraculous Work

> *It is my pleasure to tell you about the*
> *miraculous signs and wonders that*
> *the Most High God has performed for me.*
>
> **—DANIEL 4:2**

Testimonies are powerful. Testimonies give people context for how good God has been to you. When you share your story about how God has changed your life and done wonderous works, it makes others more aware of His goodness. Not everyone has accounts that they attribute to the goodness of God. You can speak of the goodness of God as a means to bring more people to Christ. Be the light, share your story, and tell people about how good God has been to you.

281 | God Still Speaks

> *I spoke to the prophets, gave them many visions, and told parables through them.*
>
> **—HOSEA 12:10**

Imagine serving a God who did not communicate with you. God communicates in various ways. God delivers life-changing messages through people, visions, and dreams. God can speak to you in such profound ways. God can provide wisdom, guidance, and direction through a powerful word of encouragement. Sometimes simply listening to a sermon or opening up your Bible provides you with a timely word from God. God is still speaking today. God spoke through the prophets, and He is still speaking through people today.

282 | Returning to God

> *"Even now," declares the* LORD, *"return to me with all your heart, with fasting and weeping and mourning."*
>
> **—JOEL 2:12**

Joel the prophet told the Israelites that despite their disobedience, God still wanted a relationship with them and that they could return to God with their hearts. This instruction is for anyone whose heart has wandered from God. Do you know someone who has drifted from their walk with Christ? Pray earnestly that they will wholeheartedly return to God and bring their troubles to Him. It is comforting to know that God will never turn us down. You or anyone who has drifted can return to God.

283 | God Desires Justice

But let justice roll on like a river, righteousness
like a never-failing stream!

—AMOS 5:24

The Bible speaks about a lack of justice for people without privileges, power, or rights. These people were often underprivileged, orphans, widows, or foreigners. Similarly, in today's world, many groups of people do not receive justice. When human systems fail to provide justice, though, God provides. God is just; He desires righteousness. When unfair treatment is rampant in the world, God sees and works on behalf of the innocent. Justice reigns supreme in Heaven. God desires justice for the innocent.

284 | Rerouting and Realigning with God

Now the LORD had arranged for a great fish
to swallow Jonah. And Jonah was inside the fish
for three days and three nights.

—JONAH 1:17

Despite Jonah's attempt to be disobedient, God orchestrated a plan to reroute Jonah and put Him back in alignment with His will. God prepared a backup plan for his mistakes. God will create a safety net when you fall. If you ever take the wrong route, God can reroute you so that you fulfill the call of God on your life. Wandering away from God's instruction can cause heartache and consequences that require prayer and deliverance. On the contrary, quick obedience offers blessings and peace.

285 | God over All

> All the nations may walk in the name of their gods, but we will walk in the name of the LORD our God for ever and ever.
>
> **—MICAH 4:5**

The world around you may choose other gods, but remain unashamed to stand boldly for God. Other people may not acknowledge Christ is Lord, you may work in contexts that do not honor God or frequent places that do not show reverence to God, but never allow the influences of the world to influence you. You can always be the one who stands out among the crowd as a Christian. Be proud to be a Citizen of Heaven and an Ambassador for Christ. You are powerful.

286 | Commonplace

> How long, LORD, must I call for help, but you do not listen? Or cry out to you, "Violence!" but you do not save?
>
> **—HABAKKUK 1:2**

Have you ever cried out to God to deliver you or fix a situation, but you felt like your requests were not heard? This is commonplace. Many people have felt this at one point or another in their lives. God answers His children in His time. He does not feel the same urgency or worry we feel because He sees the entire situation. He is not intimidated because He is in control. Everything God does is divinely orchestrated and perfectly purposed. Trust God's design.

287 | Practicing Mindfulness

> *Now this is what the* LORD *Almighty says:*
> *"Give careful thought to your ways."*
>
> **—HAGGAI 1:5**

The Israelites had given up on rebuilding God's temple and were experiencing a financial deficit because of their decision to give up. Consequences come from how we live life. We must be mindful of our ways. Carefully considering our thoughts and behaviors provides wisdom. When we are self-aware, we contribute to our development. Becoming mindful of what we give our time and energy to protects us from self-destructing, repeating poor cycles, and inhibiting our growth. Being self-aware allows us to advance.

288 | Messes into Messages

> *You intended to harm me, but God intended*
> *it for good to accomplish what is now*
> *being done, the saving of many lives.*
>
> **—GENESIS 50:20**

People may fail you and mean you harm, but God is always in control. Others may attempt to make a mess of your life, but God turns messes into messages. People may have mistreated, used, and abused you, but God can turn what they meant for evil to work for your good. God is never overpowered by someone else's poor treatment and behavior toward you. God can work all things out for your good. God's plan is greater than other people's attempt to harm you.

289 | True Love and Goodness

Love must be sincere. Hate what is evil;
cling to what is good.

—ROMANS 12:9

Love is not always easy, but it is certainly worth it. Love is patient and kind. It is authentic and genuine. Love is true affection, genuine care, and concern for others. Show love authentically. In contrast, evil is something we should hate. Hating evil means not ascribing your identity, spending time, or putting forth energy toward anything that is in direct opposition to God. Hold on to what is good, rewarding, fulfilling, and peaceful. Radiate authentic love, resist evil, and cling to goodness.

290 | Anchored Hope of the Soul

We have this hope as an anchor for the soul,
firm and secure. It enters the
inner sanctuary behind the curtain.

—HEBREWS 6:19

Hope is often referenced with an anchor in the Bible. When we consider the symbolism behind anchors, we know that they are strong and immovable. Let your hope be immovable. Let the hope in your soul be firmly planted and secure. Hope in the Lord and renew your strength. Hope in the Lord, and He will relight and restore your inner light. You may lose hope in situations, but if you ever lose hope in yourself, pull strength from the hope you have in God.

291 | God Will See You Through

> *Therefore do not worry about tomorrow,*
> *for tomorrow will worry about itself.*
> *Each day has enough trouble of its own.*
>
> **—MATTHEW 6:34**

People harbor worry, fear, and anxiety about the uncertainty of tomorrow. The truth is that tomorrow is in God's hands. Relinquish the need to control unforeseeable outcomes. Tomorrow will be what tomorrow will be. While you may not know what tomorrow holds, you can be thankful for who holds tomorrow. No matter what happens, you can trust that God will work things out for your good. The Lord will cover you with His love, protection, and grace. God will see you through anything that surfaces.

292 | Comfort in God's Promise

> *My comfort in my suffering is this:*
> *Your promise preserves my life.*
>
> **—PSALM 119:50**

When life gets tough, your comfort, hope, and peace can be found in God's promise. The Bible is filled with promises from God. Whenever you feel the heaviness of life, remember that God's promise withstands life's tests. The storms of life are often tests of your faith and hope in God's promises. Always remember that despite what happens in your life, the promises of God can and will still prevail. No test can override God's promises. God's Word to you remains the same no matter the season.

293 | Strength and Hope

Be strong and take heart, all you who hope in the LORD.

—PSALM 31:24

Be strong and take heart. When you hope in the Lord, your hope is filled. When you hope in the Lord, your faith is fueled. Rather than ruminating on hopeless thoughts, activate the strength within to remain hopeful in the Lord. Silence your fears, cast down your worries, and renew your hope through the strength God gave you. God gives us the capacity to be strong in life. Your hope in God renews your strength. To take heart means to take comfort, confidence, and control over your mind.

294 | The Power of Knowing God

Grace and peace be yours in abundance through the knowledge of God and of Jesus our LORD.

—2 PETER 1:2

Peter wanted his readers to know about the power of knowing God. To know God is to know the creator, supplier, and deliverer of grace and peace. Your knowledge of God can authorize a release of supernatural and abundant grace and peace. The joys of this world may offer temporary peace, but an Eternal God will offer you an abundance of peace and grace. This type of peace does not fade. This peace cannot be tainted. To know God is to know an eternal giver.

295 | Confidence Breeds Rich Rewards

So do not throw away your confidence;
it will be richly rewarded.

—HEBREWS 10:35

You may encounter people who are not hopeful that Jesus has come for mankind's salvation; these same people may not believe in the promises of God, but keep your confidence. This type of confidence is confidence that Jesus saves, that Jesus is, and that Jesus promises. This confidence is a belief that God's promises come to fruition because His word cannot come back void. His promises are fulfilled. This confidence is deep certainty and assuredness about Jesus. Your confidence in God will be richly rewarded.

296 | Childlike Faith

Truly I tell you, anyone who will not receive the
kingdom of God like a little child will never enter it.

—MARK 10:15

To have childlike faith is to be filled with wonder, hopeful expectation, and massive faith. The innocence of a child can teach us the value of humility, gentleness, and pure intentions. Children often have big imaginations and capacities to believe. In the same way, allow your inner child to reawaken old hopes and dreams. Walk humbly like a child and believe largely like a child. Life, complexities, and challenges may have altered the way you believe, but God desires that you keep your hope alive, youthful, and vibrant.

297 | Godly Mercy and Compassion

> This is what the LORD Almighty said: "Administer true justice; show mercy and compassion to one another."
>
> **—ZECHARIAH 7:9**

We serve a just God who believes in justice, mercy, and compassion. The measure at which we require and need justice, mercy, and compassion should be the measure we are willing to extend to others. We never know how much someone is going through or how much that person has been through. We do not know anyone's private battles and deepest pains, but we do know a God who is merciful and compassionate. We can work to be a reflection of God's loving mercy and compassion.

298 | Obedience and Blessings

> "Then all the nations will call you blessed, for yours will be a delightful land," says the LORD Almighty.
>
> **—MALACHI 3:12**

Israel struggled with obedience to God. When Israel decided to be faithful to God, God blessed them. This applies to everyone. True faithfulness and commitment to doing the right thing is rewarding. True devotion to heeding God's direction and instruction offers blessings. God loves to bless His children, but we must be in the right place to receive those blessings. We may not always do the right thing, but it does not change God's heart toward us. When we align with Him, He freely bestows blessings.

299 | God Desired a Relationship with You

For there is one God and one mediator between God and mankind, the man Christ Jesus.

—1 TIMOTHY 2:5

While people may make other things their god, there is only one God and one mediator. Jesus Christ came to Earth to take on the weight of sin and speak on your behalf to God. Jesus is the reason nothing stands in the way of your relationship with God. No sin or shortcoming is more powerful than the ultimate sacrifice that was the life of Jesus. God did not want sin to stand in the way of your salvation. He deeply desired a relationship with you.

300 | Walking in Truth

I have no greater joy than to hear that my children are walking in the truth.

—3 JOHN 1:4

This letter and compliment was intended for a Christian man named Gaius. This compliment was given to him in a time when people were more concerned with their status and reputation than walking in the truth. This is still the reality for many leaders today. Be the Christian who stands out and walks in the truth. Walking in truth honors God. Everyone may not like the truth, but the goal is not to be favored by man more than you are favored by God.

301 | Your Voice Matters

> *Be merciful to those who doubt.*
>
> **—JUDE 1:22**

There is a difference between people who scoff at Jesus and those who doubt the truth about Jesus. Being merciful to people who doubt is about having compassion for those who do not have enough clarity to believe in Jesus. Do you know your voice matters? Your testimony about Jesus matters. Your love for Jesus and the way you speak about Him matters. You may not convince every doubter, but you can bring doubters closer to the undeniable truth that God exists, and He loves everyone.

302 | What a Good God

> *"I am the Alpha and the Omega," says the LORD God,*
> *"who is, and who was, and who is to come, the Almighty."*
>
> **—REVELATION 1:8**

God is the beginning and the end. God has the whole world in His mighty hands and under His divine control. It is a blessing to have a God who is all-powerful, all-knowing, and everywhere. God is not limited or confined by natural existence. He is the creator of all things. God's divine identity provides peace and comfort. We serve a good God who is just, mighty, loving, and forgiving. We serve a God who is able to empathize and to show compassion.

303 | Letting God Steer the Ship

> *Jesus was in the stern, sleeping on a cushion. The disciples woke him and said to him, "Teacher, don't you care if we drown?"*
>
> **—MARK 4:38**

Jesus was not concerned with the storms that surfaced or any challenges the disciples faced because He would never allow the storms of life to harm them. The disciples were fearful because they were considering their circumstance from a human perspective rather than considering that they had divine help with them. In the same way, in life we often consider our storms from a natural perspective without considering that we serve a God who is omnipresent and would never leave us in any battle alone.

304 | God's Ways Are Higher

> *"For my thoughts are not your thoughts, neither are your ways my ways," declares the* LORD.
>
> **—ISAIAH 55:8**

It is a blessing that God's thoughts and His ways are higher than ours. God sees and perceives things with divine wisdom. We may see things from a limited perspective, but God sees and perceives the things we cannot. You may not always grasp what God is doing in your life, but you can trust what He is doing. God will work things out for your good. God's ways reveal His supernatural identity. His ways remind us of His power.

305 | Growing Your Blessings

Whoever can be trusted with very little can also be trusted with much, and whoever is dishonest with very little will also be dishonest with much.

—LUKE 16:10

God can and will bless you with much. Every blessing comes with some degree of responsibility. When you show God that you can faithfully manage a little, He will confidently bless you with much. When God blesses people, He blesses them with His best for their lives. When we humble ourselves to manage what we are blessed with wisely, He trusts us with more.

306 | Repentance and Holy Spirit Gifting

Peter replied, "Repent and be baptized, each of you, in the name of Jesus Christ for the forgiveness of your sins, and you will receive the gift of the Holy Spirit."

—ACTS 2:38

An outward declaration of internal faith, to repent simply means to turn away from those things that do not serve God. Asking God for forgiveness simply means acknowledging that we are not perfect but that we are humble enough to accept forgiveness from a perfect God and to open our hearts to receive the Holy Spirit. The Holy Spirit provides you with wisdom, discernment, and clarity. God does not require perfection from you; He simply desires your love, devotion, and commitment.

307 | You Are Valuable

Through him all things were made; without him nothing was made that has been made.

—JOHN 1:3

God is the Creator of the Universe. Nothing that occurs in the world is out of His reach. You can be confident that God knows what is happening in the world He created. He sees all things. The world may not be a reflection of what His initial plan for peace was, but you are. You are valuable and your existence in the purposeful world He created matters. God created your very existence, and He wants you to walk boldly in your identity in Christ.

308 | God Grants Peace

The LORD turn his face toward you and give you peace.

—NUMBERS 6:26

Peace is comfort in knowing that, though you may not have control over what has happened or what will happen in your life, God is with you. Peace is being secure in the fact that God's love for you outweighs the difficulties in life. You may struggle and face hardships, but God will grant you peace despite the storm. Peace is assuredness that all things work together for good for those that love the Lord and for those who are called according to His purpose.

309 | God Reigns Supreme

> *The* LORD *reigns, let the earth be glad; let the distant shores rejoice.*
>
> **—PSALM 97:1**

God reigns supreme over your life, your finances, your health, your relationships, and your children. God has a destiny plan over your life. It may not look like blessings are coming your way but God reigns supreme. It may not look like God is working, but God reigns supreme. He is supreme in power, all-forgiving, all-loving, and never-ending. God reigns supreme over the world. He has the final say. God will never fail. Rejoice! You are covered by the God who reigns supreme.

310 | Kindness Toward Others

> *Be wise in the way you act toward outsiders; make the most of every opportunity.*
>
> **—COLOSSIANS 4:5**

People should feel God's loving, merciful, forgiving, and just character. He is holy and to be revered, but He's not legalistic and dominating over His children. Thus, when you make the declaration that you are Christian, you are identifying with His love, grace, and mercy. Let your treatment of others be a reflection of God. Make the most of every opportunity to be kind, gentle, loving, caring, and forgiving. People need their hope restored in the kindness of humanity and the love of Jesus Christ.

311 | God Heals All Hearts

The LORD is close to the brokenhearted and saves those who are crushed in spirit.

—PSALM 34:18

Even when you feel misunderstood in your brokenness, God understands. God is near the brokenhearted. He saves those whose spirits have been crushed. There is not a broken heart God cannot heal; there is not a crushed spirit He cannot mend. The matters of your heart concern God. He cares for you. Your life and the experiences you have are important to God. He desires to hear from you. He wants to comfort you and to bring you through those tough places.

312 | Seeking God's Face

Look to the LORD and his strength; seek his face always.

—PSALM 105:4

God's strength is greater than our own. To have access to His strength is to experience an abundance of willpower, tenacity, and the ability to handle life. Seeking the Lord's face in everything provides for supernatural strength and wisdom. When you seek God's face, you receive clarity. While you may not always know the right direction to go, relying on God offers you divine direction, wisdom, and guidance. No matter the season, strength and guidance from God are valuable. Seek God's face, and rely on His strength.

313 | He Never Forsakes You

> *Those who know your name trust in you, for you, LORD,*
> *have never forsaken those who seek you.*
>
> **—PSALM 9:10**

When you know God's name, you perceive the power His name holds. The name of the Lord is above every other name. His name is an active change agent. Things change when we say His name. The atmosphere shifts when we declare His glory. God's name changes the trajectory of your life. He never forsakes those who trust Him and call on His name. When you call on His name, no battle or tough season can overpower you. The name of the Lord breeds power.

314 | Humbly Valuing Others

> *Do nothing out of selfish ambition or vain conceit.*
> *Rather, in humility value others above yourselves.*
>
> **—PHILIPPIANS 2:3**

Sometimes we are consumed with personal needs and desires, but valuable relationships require our attention. Whenever we shift our focus off of ourselves and onto the needs of those we love, we operate from a place of humility. This does not mean that you should neglect and ignore your needs; rather, you have the opportunity to share the love your harbor within, with others. Humbly value your relationships. God gives you your people for a reason. He entrusts you with loving them right.

> *And will not God bring about justice for his chosen ones, who cry out to him day and night? Will he keep putting them off?*
>
> **—LUKE 18:7**

Have you ever experienced a situation that only God could solve? In this biblical account, a widow needed a judge to grant her justice in her case. This judge did not fear God or care about people. The judge ruled in her favor because the widow was persistent. Have the kind of faith that frustrates the enemy. Pray so consistently that God moves the hearts of the unloving. Pray and believe so much in your justice that it is granted because of God's favor over your life. Sometimes the natural circumstances of your life look like you will not make it out, but God, God is an all-of-a-sudden God, who shows up and shows out for you. Your life circumstances may not look favorable, but God can do the unthinkable for you. This judge was not inclined to grant this woman justice, but her persistence frustrated his normal response to people. Persistence is a result of faith at work. She had so much faith that it worked out for her in the end.

Live Out the Word

What is your heart's hope? Journal about the things you lost hope in or that you have been hoping for. Pray about it daily. Trust God.

316 | Take in God's Word

> *Consequently, faith comes from hearing the message,
> and the message is heard through the word about Christ.*
>
> **—ROMANS 10:17**

Faith is built through prayer, Bible reading, listening to
sound doctrine, and praise and worship. Life experiences
can catapult one's faith to great heights or substantially
compromise one's faith. Most important is the active imple-
mentation of taking in God's Word. God's Word provides
clarity about the promises He's made you, the way He views
you, and His character. Understanding the characteristics
of God offers confidence in how He operates in situations.
When life experiences surface, people either lean into their
faith or fall away from their faith. When you read the Word,
you understand that God may not always come when you
want Him to, but He is always on time. When you read the
Word, you understand that weeping may endure for a night,
but joy comes in the morning. When you read the Word, you
understand that God will never leave nor forsake you. It is
vital to one's faith to hear the word and the messages of
God. Though Faith can be strengthened in many ways, the
Bible is a main source.

Live Out the Word

Challenge yourself to read the Bible, listen to a sermon, and
journal about what you learn every day. Testify about how it
affects your faith.

317 | Your Life Reflects Your Heart

As water reflects the face, so one's life reflects the heart.

—PROVERBS 27:19

Your life is often a reflection of your heart's condition. If you value work, then the benefits of working are reflected in your life; if your heart is your kids, then your kids reflect that love and care. If you value love, peace, and joy, those things radiate more fluidly in your life. If your heart is filled with envy, sadness, and bitterness, your life will exude those things. Wherever you want your life to improve, study and examine your heart's condition and work to improve accordingly.

318 | Ability and Confidence from God

Not that we are competent in ourselves to claim any-thing for ourselves, but our competence comes from God.

—2 CORINTHIANS 3:5

Imposter syndrome is the false belief that you are under-qualified and not knowledgeable enough or skilled enough for the field that you have skills and expertise in. We psych ourselves out of performing when we rely too heavily on our own abilities. To rely on your skills is to depend on your confidence to be consistent enough to perform the skill. When you rely on God to perform, your confidence is rooted in the God who gave you your gifts and your confidence is less likely to waver.

319 | Follow God, Lose the World

What good will it be for someone to gain the whole world, yet forfeit their soul? Or what can anyone give in exchange for their soul?

—MATTHEW 16:26

Following Jesus is an internal decision that should be reflected in your external habits. When the disciples followed Jesus, they left behind their homes, families, and professions. Deciding to follow Jesus requires sacrifice. You may never have to leave your home and family to follow Him, but you must often forsake old habits and decide against following the world. Sacrifice is a common experience for believers. It is far better to sacrifice worldly acceptance than it is to sacrifice a real relationship with God.

320 | Genuine Gain for Self-Improvement

And I saw that all toil and all achievement spring from one person's envy of another. This too is meaningless, a chasing after the wind.

—ECCLESIASTES 4:4

When you are pursuing a dream or working hard toward a goal, consider your heart's intention. Always seek to pursue your goals and dreams to improve upon the last version of yourself. True gain is that which stems from genuine intentions, hard work, and effort. The most rewarding gain comes from a natural desire to improve rather than to compare and compete.

321 | Success for the Upright

He holds success in store for the upright, he is a shield to those whose walk is blameless.

—PROVERBS 2:7

Success is not confined to monetary contentment. Success also means a happy, healthy, and positive home life. What a joy it is to know that God holds success for those who try to lead honest lives. That means He reserves successful encounters, divine connections, and supernatural doors of alignment for your destiny. God keeps you in mind and works behind the scenes to ensure your success. God is a shield to those whose walk is blameless. When you honor God with your life, He blesses you.

322 | Becoming the Righteousness of God

God made him who had no sin to be sin for us, so that in him we might become the righteousness of God.

—2 CORINTHIANS 5:21

Jesus was perfect, blameless, and without sin, yet He took on the cross for the salvation of mankind. He became the sacrifice for our sins so that we might become the righteousness of God. Becoming the righteousness of God is to be in Christ. When we walk with Christ, we reflect God's love for mankind. Jesus bore the weight of mankind's wrongs because of the overwhelming love God has for us. God's love for us was sacrificial. Sometimes our love for Him requires sacrificing poor lifestyle habits.

323 | An Unchanging and Merciful God

> *The LORD is good to all, and his mercy is over all that he has made.*
>
> **—PSALM 145:9**

God is good no matter what. The Lord is good whether the circumstances appear favorable or not. Sometimes people endure hardship and blame God and view Him negatively. God does not change just because our life situations change. He remains loving, compassionate, and just. He is a merciful God who does not want harm to come to His children. No matter what happens in life, God is still good. He has not forgotten you; He loves you unconditionally, and you matter a great deal to Him.

324 | A Light to My Path

> *Your word is a lamp for my feet, and a light to my path.*
>
> **—PSALM 119:105**

The Word of God illuminates the path of your destiny. God's Word provides insight and clarity that the world cannot. God's Word illuminates dark places and leads you along the right path. Life may feel confusing sometimes; doors open and uncertainty about which route to go may surface, but God's Word aligns you with truth. The path that reflects God's will is ultimately the best path to take. When you are unsure, you can find enlightenment in God's Word. God's Word is filled with promise.

325 | Lacking Nothing

Those who seek the LORD lack no good thing.

—PSALM 34:10

Seeking God fills you. Seeking God completes you internally. God will point out areas in you that need healing and work with you to mend those areas. He will supply any needs you have. He will fill your empty spaces. If you lack emotional support, He will support you emotionally. If you lack love, He will love you unconditionally. If you lack care, He will care for you eternally. God is a filler of empty space and areas of unfulfillment. With God, you lack nothing.

326 | Everlasting Covenant

Yet I will remember the covenant I made with you in the days of your youth, and I will establish an everlasting covenant with you.

—EZEKIEL 16:60

It is a relief to know that God remembers the promises He makes to us. This promise was pertaining to Israel. Despite their disobedience to God, God's merciful forgiveness would be the reason for the fulfillment of God's promises to the nation. Similarly, it is not by any acts of righteousness but by God's grace that He remembers the promises He makes with you and keeps His word. His everlasting covenant with you is rooted in His love and gracious mercy for you.

327 | The Unseen vs. the Seen

> *So we fix our eyes not on what is seen, but on what is unseen, since what is seen is temporary, but what is unseen is eternal.*
>
> **—2 CORINTHIANS 4:18**

Paul reflects in this Scripture on his refusal to lose faith that God will see him through tough times. Sometimes we are fixated on the natural circumstances rather than focusing on the supernatural. If we fix our eyes on what is seen, we lose focus on the eternal, which is God. God is more powerful; He is the ultimate problem solver. It is far better to fix your focus on the problem solver rather than the problem. Focusing on the problem increases worry and doubt. Focus on God; trust God.

328 | The Lord Watches over You

> *The LORD will keep you from all harm—he will watch over your life; the LORD will watch over your coming and going both now and forevermore.*
>
> **—PSALM 121:7-8**

How comforting is it to know that God watches over you? He cares enough about you to safeguard you from hurt, harm, and danger. God will protect you from danger seen and unseen. He will keep you safeguarded and protected by His holy angels. God cares for your well-being. Your life matters to God. He covers you; He will protect you from evil and all things not meant for you.

329 | Being Content in All Seasons

I am not saying this because I am in need, for I have learned to be content whatever the circumstances.

—PHILIPPIANS 4:11

Paul learned to be content in any situation because He understood that God would see Him through anything. You may feel like you do not have a way out, but God is not always concerned with pulling you out as much as he wants to pull you through tough situations. In tough seasons, you grow while God grooms. Tough seasons give you wisdom, foster resilience, and compel you to total reliance on God.

330 | Live Actively in God's Word

But the seed on good soil stands for those with a noble and good heart, who hear the word, retain it, and by persevering produce a crop.

—LUKE 8:15

It is not enough to simply know the Word; we must apply the Word to our lives. You experience a real breakthrough then. Even the enemy knows God's Word, so real power comes from actively living God's Word. It is most important to retain the Word and apply it to your life. God's power is revealed in your life through active faith and application of biblical principles.

331 | Do Things with God

Unless the LORD builds the house, the builders labor in vain. Unless the LORD watches over the city, the guards stand watch in vain.

—PSALM 127:1

Do things with God instead of consulting Him in the aftermath. Waiting on God's acceptance for your next endeavor provides peace and confidence. When you decide before talking with God, you run the risk of making ill-informed decisions that impact your life adversely. Go to God, get insight, and then build. Unless the Lord is spearheading your decisions, you may be working in vain. Working in vain may put you two steps back rather than catapulting your life in the right direction. Go to God first.

332 | Children of God

See what great love the Father has lavished on us, that we should be called children of God!

—1 JOHN 3:1

It is a privilege to be called a Child of God. God could have called us His imperfect creations, but He wanted us to be His children. He wanted us to be in divine relationship with Him. God's love for you is so vast that you do not fully perceive its magnitude. God loves you the way good parents love their children, authentically, without limits, and unconditionally. His love for you does not waver. You are His child when you mess up and even when people reject you.

333 | Search My Heart

*Search me, God, and know my heart; test me
and know my anxious thoughts.*

—PSALM 139:23

David was a man after God's own heart, but he was an imperfect man after God's heart. He asked God to search his heart so he could do away with sin and poor habits. David wanted to lead an honest life, walk upright, and serve the Lord. In the same way, you may be doing your best as a Christian, but asking God to search you and make you aware of those things that you should part ways with helps you to improve and develop.

334 | Keep Reaching God's People

*All this is for your benefit, so that the grace that is
reaching more and more people may cause thanksgiving
to overflow to the glory of God.*

—2 CORINTHIANS 4:15

Spreading the Gospel can come with a lot of sacrifice. Paul endured hardship in order to keep preaching the Gospel. His work was not in vain, and neither is yours. Whatever work you commit to, let it reflect your faith. Whatever sacrifices you make to model ministry in your work, know that it reaches people. People need the work you do for the Lord. Ministry can be found in any profession. Keep walking in your calling, serving others, and reaching people for God.

> *We are therefore Christ's ambassadors, as though God were making his appeal through us. We implore you on Christ's behalf: Be reconciled to God.*
>
> **—2 CORINTHIANS 5:20**

Evangelism is vital to the Kingdom of God. An ambassador for Jesus is someone who cares for people's salvation. Making your life's work about getting more people saved is Kingdom work. It does not matter what professional calling you have; you can use that calling to spread the Gospel. People need to know that Jesus loves them. People need to know that Heaven is possible for them. Sometimes God puts you in places with certain people so that you can introduce them to Jesus. No matter the professional title, make saving souls a top priority on your list of obligations. Evangelism is not a choice that Jesus left us to make. Evangelism is the mandate that Jesus left the disciples. It did not matter whether they were educated or formal in their delivery, it only mattered that they were committed to sharing the good news with lost souls. Similarly, God is relying on you to share the good news. You are capable and qualified enough to share your faith with others. Your evangelism can save lives.

Live Out the Word

Challenge yourself to talk to three people this week about the good news. These should be people you know or lost, or complete strangers.

336 | Endurance Produces Character

> *Suffering produces perseverance; perseverance, character; and character, hope.*
>
> **—ROMANS 5:3–4**

Every good work and successful endeavor will require endurance. Endurance is the desire to push past any limiting beliefs and blockages in order to meet goals. Enduring tough seasons helps you to build confidence, character, and resilience. Endurance is the ability to keep persisting despite how tough a season can be. Many of your tough seasons that require endurance build your character in a way that is conducive to your future blessings.

337 | Contentment with Basic Provision

> *But if we have food and clothing, we will be content with that.*
>
> **—1 TIMOTHY 6:8**

We may not always get what we want, but we can thank God for meeting our needs. Paul spoke about being content with having personal needs met. This is not to be confused with thinking having nice things is wrong; it is simply that nice things should not consume you. Never be consumed with things that are not God. Being content with what you have and the needs that God meets is an expression of gratitude.

338 | Love Correctly

> *[Love] always protects, always trusts,*
> *always hopes, always perseveres.*
>
> **—1 CORINTHIANS 13:7**

Paul spoke about what love should and should not be. Loving like God loves is not easy. God's love reflects the qualities Paul speaks about. The standard of love was meant to be applied to God, ourselves, and others. The truth is, some of the people we love do not know how to love. We can experience pain from rejection, harm, and mistreatment from those we love. It is important to know that this is never okay. It is one thing to decide to love someone through thick and thin despite the other person doing things that annoy you; it is an entirely different thing to love someone who mistreats you. God never intended for love to cause harm. God wants you to know love that is present for you, supports you, genuinely cares for you, believes in you, and protects you. If someone claims to love you but consistently harms you, their definition of love is unhealthy and not biblical. Always seek to protect your mind, body, and spirit. Your well-being matters. Love should reflect God.

Live Out the Word

How can we love ourselves and others the way God loves? Including yourself, list the people you want to actively love on this week.

339 | Thankful for a Supernatural God

> *God is not human, that he should lie, not a human being, that he should change his mind. Does he speak and then not act? Does he promise and not fulfill?*
>
> **—NUMBERS 23:19**

It is truly a blessing that God relates to His children but does not possess human tendencies. God does not lie. What He declares manifests. What He orders and directs comes to fruition. God is not capable of deceiving you. He decides in His mind about His love for you and the promises He has in store for you. He does not change His mind about you. Whatever He promises, He follows through on. We serve a faithful God. Be thankful that God is supernatural.

340 | Protect Your Peace

> *Do not be misled: "Bad company corrupts good character."*
>
> **—1 CORINTHIANS 15:33**

Paul was warning the believers to be watchful so as not to be misled by those who did not believe in the resurrection of Jesus. Paul warned against comingling with people who freely sin and disregard God's divine design. In the same way, it is crucial to your mental and spiritual health that you analyze the company you keep. Not all company is good company. Your spiritual and mental life can be impacted by those who freely practice sin. Protect your peace and safeguard your space.

341 | God Cares for Everyone

> On hearing this, Jesus said to them, "It is not
> the healthy who need a doctor, but the sick. I have
> not come to call the righteous, but sinners."
>
> **—MARK 2:17**

Jesus came for those who needed healing most. He came
for those in need of physical healing and heart healing. As
Christians, we may not be able to mingle with just anyone,
but we can certainly pray for everyone. We can pray for
people to experience a change of heart toward God. There
are broken and hurting people who hurt others because
they need God's healing hand over their lives. We can
pray for total healing and restoration for people who have
been exposed to life's greatest pains. We can pray for the
unbeliever, the hostile neighbor, and the angry coworker.
Everyone needs prayer. As Christians, we should be willing
to pray for people who do not look like us, live like us, act
like us, believe like us, and speak like us. We must be the
light God called us to be. We may be the only Christian that
people encounter in their daily lives. The need for us to be
the light and remain diligent in prayer is great.

Live Out the Word

Write down a list of people who need prayer. These should
be people you never or seldom pray for. Pray for each
listed person.

342 | Let God Be the Judge

*It is God who judges: He brings one down,
he exalts another.*

—PSALM 75:7

Judgment is a critical perception about someone else's life. It has never been our place to judge. Our place is to love people. We do not know someone else's life story. You may not agree with how someone does things, but God ultimately has the final say and He issues just judgments to each person. It is no one's place to judge you either. God judges each person accordingly. Tend to your life, pray for others, and love them as God would have you do.

343 | God Strengthens Hearts

*My flesh and my heart may fail, but God is the
strength of my heart and my portion forever.*

—PSALM 73:26

This passage refers to Asaph, who was upset with God because he did not understand what God was doing in his life. Asaph later settles his discontentment and asserts that God is important to him. This feeling of uneasiness about God's ways is commonplace. Humans make mistakes, fail, and fall short, but God remains your strength. God will pull you through anything. God has plans to prosper and grow you. He cares about your life and your future. He does not mean you any harm.

344 | Small but Mighty

The least of you will become a thousand,
the smallest a mighty nation. I am the LORD;
in its time I will do this swiftly.

—ISAIAH 60:22

Israel was a small nation, but at God's appointed time, He strengthened Israel. Israel became a nation that was mighty and strong. In the same way, you may feel like you are but one person on a big mission. Maybe your dreams and goals are far bigger than yourself, but at God's appointed time, He will strengthen you and make you mighty among the larger names in your field. God is not incapable of promoting you and placing you in a place of authority.

345 | Cheerful Giver

Each of you should give what you have decided
in your heart to give, not reluctantly or
under compulsion, for God loves a cheerful giver.

—2 CORINTHIANS 9:7

Paul was speaking of giving financial resources, though all giving should be done with a cheerful heart. If you are giving tithes and offerings, do so cheerfully. If it is quality time you extend to someone in need of companionship, do so cheerfully. If it is a resource you offer someone who is lacking, do so cheerfully. The moral of the message is, when you give, whether it is monetary or anything of value, it should prompt your humility in a way that makes God's heart smile.

346 | Stop Playing Small

If you remain in me and my words remain in you, ask whatever you wish, and it will be done for you.

—JOHN 15:7

Many people doubt what they can do on Earth because they do not realize the power in aligning with God and becoming the fullness of all they were intended to be. Some people play small because it feels safe. Though, if you remain in God and His Word remains in you, what you ask God for can come to life. You do not have to be timid, and you do not have to play small. What is for you God will bring to pass.

347 | Trust God and Do Good

Trust the LORD and do good; live in the land, and farm faithfulness.

—PSALM 37:3

Trust God, do good in the world, and whatever work you commit to doing, do so faithfully. Whatever your work is, do it to your best ability and trust God through it all. Your work may be hard, exhausting, or extremely time-consuming, but God sees the honest work you are putting in. God is not oblivious to all that you do. Continue to trust God to get you through the challenging days. Lean on God for discernment and clarity about how to navigate your work.

348 | God Is Always Trustworthy

Trust in the Lord forever, for the Lord, the Lord himself, is the Rock eternal.

—ISAIAH 26:4

You can trust God in every season of your life. In good seasons, trust that God wants you to walk into His very best for you. In your low seasons, trust that God has a plan for you and that He makes all things work for your good. The Rock is God. He was rejected, but He is undefeated. God is reliable in every season. People may come in and out of your life, but God is trustworthy and reliable in all of your seasons.

349 | Let Your Faith Be Loud

You see that a person is considered righteous by what they do and not by faith alone.

—JAMES 2:24

Faith supported with actions is a force to be reckoned with. Your faith should be loud. This means your life should reflect your faith. Faith is doing things for your future despite feeling afraid. Faith is doing your part while waiting for God to do His. Faith should be the leading force that dominates any fear you feel. Let your faith be louder than your fear. Make decisions that reflect faith in God. Faith in action is taking bold steps despite having uncertainty about the outcome.

350 | Humility and Servitude

For even the Son of Man did not come to be served, but to serve, and to give his life as a ransom for many.

—MATTHEW 20:28

Jesus was not born into a rich family, nor was He dressed in royal clothes. He certainly did not live in mansions. Jesus was a carpenter. He was from a town that was not considered popular or attractive. Jesus walked this Earth as a human being with an average life. Jesus was humble. He was royalty born as ordinary. Jesus did not come to be served; He came to serve people. He gave His life for you. Let humility promote your servitude for others.

351 | God Gets the Glory

But we have this treasure in jars of clay to show that this all-surpassing power is from God and not from us.

—2 CORINTHIANS 4:7

Paul acknowledged that God's glory shining through him gave him abilities. We must give God glory for the greatness that comes from us. God's supernatural power working through us produces confidence. It is not by our might that we are strong; it is by God's might. We must believe in the power of God working through us. Paul made many strides in ministry, but he knew that if it were not for the power of God, he would not be capable of such great strides.

352 | God the Redeemer

> *I know that you can do all things; no purpose*
> *of yours can be thwarted.*

—JOB 42:2

Job understood that he was a sinful man, but that God was a redeemer. Job's whole world came crashing down in just one day. Job maintained His respect for God and spoke to God's sovereignty. God can do anything and make anything happen in just a moment's time. God's work cannot be over-ridden. If you have been experiencing backlash, oppression, rejection, pain, and discontentment, know that God is still good. God sees you and cares. God is never limited. He is omnipotent.

353 | Deserving of a Beautiful Life

> *The thief comes only to steal and kill and destroy; I have*
> *come that they may have life, and have it to the full.*

—JOHN 10:10

God wants you to have access to His best. God desires for you to experience quality relationships and heart-filling experiences. God wants you to see the fulfillment of the hopes and dreams He has placed in your heart. When you encounter a stolen dream, a hope killed, or a dismantled belief, you can attribute that to the enemy attempting to stand in the way of you enjoying a beautiful and fulfilling life. The enemy cannot dismantle what God has deemed possible for your life.

354 | God Is Love

> Whoever does not love does not know God,
> because God is love.
>
> **—1 JOHN 4:8**

Work to make love your top characteristic. God is love. In
fact, He so loved us that He wrapped His Son in flesh and
offered Him as a sacrifice to atone for sin. Christians are
sinners saved by grace. We are flawed but loved. Thus, we
must be willing to humbly extend grace and love to others.
Everyone is on a different level of awareness about God.
Show people love and grace, and you will show them God.
Walking in love is walking with God.

355 | A God That Understands

> For we do not have a high priest who is unable to
> empathize with our weaknesses, but we
> have one who has been tempted in every way,
> just as we are—yet he did not sin.
>
> **—HEBREWS 4:15**

We serve a God who fully understands how difficult it can
be to rise above the challenges of temptation. He empathizes with mankind. God never allows us to be tempted
beyond what we can manage. When we are tempted, He
always provides a way out of the temptation. The next time
you are tempted, ask God to show you how to rise above
the temptation, He will help you overcome the temptation
to sin. Remember, temptation is not stronger than God's
love for you.

356 | Strength and Peace from God

> *The LORD gives strength to his people;*
> *the LORD blesses his people with peace.*
>
> **—PSALM 29:11**

The Lord strengthens His people. He is compassionate, loving, and caring. His children mean a great deal to Him. God blesses His children with peace. Do you perceive the magnitude of God's care and concern for you? Do you know that He hears your prayers and deeply yearns to have a relationship with you? God is not distant to your heart. No matter the season, God equips you with strength and offers you His peace.

357 | Give According to Your Ability

> *Each of you must bring a gift in proportion to the*
> *way the LORD your God has blessed you.*
>
> **—DEUTERONOMY 16:17**

While not everyone has the same capacity to give, always give what you can. God is a giver and expects us to be givers. You can never outgive and outdo God. That means when you give to others, God can bless you and give you more giving capacity. Giving is an opportunity for God to bless others through you. God blesses givers. God is a giver and loves when His children freely give. Give what you can, and God will use your giving for His glory.

358 | God Shows No Favoritism

> *Then Peter began to speak: "I now realize how true it is that God does not show favoritism."*
>
> **—ACTS 10:34**

God does not show favoritism to His children. You may feel like God blesses someone more than He blesses you, but God does not value one child over the other. God loves His children equally. God wants a relationship with the sinner as much as He wants to be in relationship with the saint. God loves the one who does not know Him yet, and the one who already does. His love is vast and unconditional. He wants every person to enter the Kingdom of Heaven.

359 | Share the Gospel Anyway

> *I came to you in weakness with great fear and trembling.*
>
> **—1 CORINTHIANS 2:3**

Paul reminds the Corinthians of his first encounters with them. Paul was not the best speaker when he initially came to the Corinthians to spread the good news of the Gospel. Paul did not attempt to appear formally educated or advanced, he simply wanted to tell them about Jesus. In the same way, it does not matter how many professional degrees or experiences you have, sharing the Gospel is for every believer to take part in. People admire relatability and clearly conveyed messages.

360 | Never Fear

> *When I am afraid, I put my trust in you.*
>
> **—PSALM 56:3**

Fear is formed to keep you from doing the next big thing in your life, taking a leap of faith, or trusting God. When you feel fear, rely on God's certainty, strength, and abilities. When you feel fear, do not rely on your human reasoning but trust in the Lord's supernatural ways. God knows the beginning and end of all things. Walk with God and allow Him to lead you. When you rely on God, you never have to fear the outcome of anything.

361 | Trust God over Everything

> *Some trust in chariots and some in horses,*
> *but we trust in the name of the LORD our God.*
>
> **—PSALM 20:7**

The world around us may trust in the creations of God rather than in God, but make a declaration of commitment to God. Be bold in your faith and know that God honors your stance. Keep being the light. Keep trusting in God, standing your ground, and speaking up when necessary about who God is. Do not waver in your trust. You know in your deepest distress that you can call on God and count on Him. You understand that His very name has power.

362 | Keep Calm

> *If a ruler's anger rises against you, do not leave your*
> *post; calmness can lay great offenses to rest.*
>
> **—ECCLESIASTES 10:4**

Solomon taught that remaining calm despite someone else's hostility can settle the conflict. In our lives, we will encounter people who are hostile and speak ill toward us. We have a choice about how we want to respond to poor interactions and offenses. We can either meet people on a lower level of operating and return the hostility, or we can rise to a higher operating version of ourselves and display humility and compassion. Wisdom eases offenses. Remaining calm displays great wisdom and self-control.

363 | Honest Gain and Good Intentions

> *Better the little that the righteous have than the*
> *wealth of many wicked; for the power of the wicked*
> *will be broken, but the* Lord *upholds the righteous.*
>
> **—PSALM 37:16-17**

God honors those who conduct business honestly. He respects honest gain and values proper handling of financial resources. It is better to have a little and to be righteous than it is to have more but have an evil heart. God is focused on the intentions of our hearts. Those who gain dishonestly or who have a lot but are evil have stored-up treasures on Earth but not in Heaven. Keep being honest, genuine, and well-intentioned. Whatever you have God will bless.

364 | Overpowering Negative People with God

In God, whose word I praise—in God I trust and am not afraid. What can mere mortals do to me?

—PSALM 56:4

Despite what people do and the negative things they say about you, they cannot overpower God. Remain confident that when people stand against you; God still stands with you. Never fear the power of man more than you acknowledge the presence of God. God sees all things and will protect you according to your need. You may walk into workplaces with poor organizational culture or frequent a church where you feel unaccepted, but trust God to vindicate you in their midst. Do not fear man; you have God.

365 | Unswerving and Unrelenting Faith

Let us hold unswervingly to the hope we profess, for he who promised is faithful.

—HEBREWS 10:23

When troubles arise, and when life happens, hold on to hope. Do not fall away from the faith. You may be tempted to doubt God or to grow angry with His timing, but trust God and fear not. He has got you covered and in the palm of His mighty hands. God will deliver on His promises to you. Despite what the circumstances appear to be, God is with you, He hears you and He cares for you. Trust God in all seasons.

Index

Acknowledgments

First, all honor, glory, and praise to God in Heaven for guiding me as I wrote this devotional. Thanks to my husband, Aaron, and my son, Elijah, for being patient with me as I stayed up late every night and missed family games and movie time to work on this project. Thanks, Callisto team, for helping me bring this dream to fruition. Thanks to my social media family for always believing in me.

About the Author

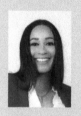 **Dr. India Logan** is a wife, mother, Christian life coach, educator, public speaker, and writer.
She runs a Christian life coaching business and a virtual Christian coaching school. She helps women develop spiritually, personally, and professionally, while specializing in singleness, motherhood, marriage, relationships, healing, healthy boundaries, and goal attainment.

Dr. India speaks at events, universities, and churches. She creates funny, educational, and inspirational Christian content on social media. Learn more at DoctorIndiaLogan.com.

In her free time, Dr. India travels the world and reads.